Ditch the Junk, Find Your Spunk

Ditch the Junk, Find Your Spunk

Tackle the Obstacles in Your Life &
Learn How to Live Abundantly

Shellby Winget, SLP, CHC, CPT

• • •

This book is dedicated to all of my thyroid peeps as well as everyone who has endured obstacles on their journey to health and wellness. I hope that my story will be a beacon of light for you and help inspire you as you strive toward total wellness. My desire is that you are able to reclaim your health and live life abundantly. Blessings!

• • •

Disclaimer

The contents of this book are the personal testimony and beliefs of the author and are meant for educational and informational purposes only. The author does not claim to be a physician, healthcare professional, registered dietitian, or expert in the healthcare field. As a certified Health Coach and Personal Trainer, it is the author's desire to motivate and inspire you to make healthy choices. However, she also wants to encourage you to make your own health and dietary decisions based upon proper research, and in partnership with your trusted healthcare provider. These tips, opinions, and writings are not intended to diagnose, treat, or cure any health problems. This information is not meant to replace your doctor's recommendations or the advice of other qualified healthcare professionals. Always check with your doctor before making any changes to your health protocol. Lastly, the information provided within this book is believed to be true and accurate;

however, the reader should assume all responsibility for consulting with his/her doctor regarding any health matter. The author and publisher deny any liability, loss, or injury in relationship with any opinion or tip shared in this book.

Acknowledgements

First, I want to thank my heavenly Father for prompting me to write this book...and helping me along the way. This was a great application of Philippians 4:13, "I can do all this through him who gives me strength." I have had so much information floating around in my head that it was hard at times to know what to include, and what to leave out. So, I spent a lot of time praying for wisdom regarding the information that would be the most useful to share.

Next, I want to thank my family for being patient with me as I occasionally had days that I didn't get around to making dinner because I was making good progress on writing this book. Plus, I am extremely grateful for their love and support. I especially want to thank my husband for not only allowing me to take time to write this book, but for encouraging me to do so. I think he thought I should have written my story several years ago. However, I'm glad that I have had additional experiences over this past year that have taught me a great deal about truly being healthy. I consider myself extremely blessed to have such an amazing husband and wonderful, caring boys. Plus, they were good sports when I made them begin an experiment on hugging (which I mention in the *Ditch the Stress* chapter), which I believe helped them as much as it did me. Thank you for your love, encouragement, and support! I love you!!!

To all my friends and family who prayed for me or encouraged me along the way...thank you! I cannot name every single person who has lifted me up, but I never could have written this book without the support of friends. No word of encouragement went unnoticed. Your words propelled me to keep going. I hope that my book will bless you as much as your words have blessed me. Thank you friends!

I am thankful for the help of two amazing doctors. First, Dr. David Boynton, DC, CCEP was originally recommended to our family to help our youngest son. However, once we got to know him, our entire family saw the value in his treatment and we all started seeing him. Dr. Boynton has helped our son make some significant gains with his gut issues. Plus, he helped me to discover the underlying issue of Candida, etc. and put me on a protocol to support it. It set me on a path to learn many new things about our microbiome. We appreciate you, Dr. Boynton!

Last, but not least, I want to express my extreme gratitude to Dr. Lauri Nandyal, MD, NCMP. In my search for a new doctor who was knowledgeable about functional endocrinology, I discovered Dr. Nandyal. She has been great at looking at the full picture in order to help me discover the underlying issues with all of my symptoms. Plus, she was very thorough at examining all of the data (both personal symptoms and lab results) and talking it through with my husband and me. Between making an adjustment to my thyroid medication and helping me discover my food intolerances...and what was going on in my gut, she has helped me regain a healthy balance to my system. You rock, Dr. Nandyal! Thanks for helping me regain my health!

Table of Contents

Disclaimer.. xi

Acknowledgements ix

Introduction... xv

Chapter 1: DO Take Care of YOU!...................................... 1

Chapter 2: Ditch the TSH Only Lab Testing.......................... 5

Chapter 3: Ditch the Endocrine Disruptors 13

Chapter 4: Ditch Food Intolerances & Antinutrients........... 21

Chapter 5: Ditch One Size Fits All Diets 37

Chapter 6: Ditch the Gunk in Your Gut 47

Chapter 7: Ditch Imbalances 69

Chapter 8: Ditch the Low Energy.. 97

Chapter 9: Ditch the Stress 105

Chapter 10: Ditch the Stinkin' Thinkin' 113

Chapter 11: My Biggest Game Changers........................... 119

Appendix A: Additional Information on Endocrine
Disruptors.. 129

Appendix B: Recommended Labs & Optimal Lab Values.. 131

Appendix C: Additional Resources 135

Appendix D: My Favorite People/Pages to Follow 139

References 145

About the Author.. 149

Introduction

My original plan in writing this book was to help others who have struggled with hypothyroidism to gain their life back. However, I have come to realize that it's not just those of us who have dealt with a sluggish thyroid (or lack of thyroid) who desire to find the answers, but many people are searching for answers to energy and weight loss. Although, after everything that I've learned over the past sixteen plus years, my guess would be that many more people suffer from thyroid issues than what is currently diagnosed. So, if you are struggling with decreased energy, weight gain, or just have lost your spunk (regardless of whether it is from thyroid issues or not), then this book is for you!

First, let me give you a little background about myself...and you will soon learn why I have a passion for helping others who struggle with energy and controlling their weight. My journey with the thyroid started almost seventeen years ago, but first I want to take you back to my youth. I essentially grew up on a farm and we had a large yard, so I had plenty of opportunities to be active. So, for me the biggest culprit was the food I was eating. I was a picky eater, and I never would have imagined eating the foods that I now eat today. I probably would have turned my nose up and outright refused to eat them. However, it's amazing how our taste buds can change (and, yes...yours can too). I literally have done a 180 in the foods that I now eat from what I used to eat when I was younger. Therefore, if I suggest eating certain types of food later on in this book, I ask that you keep an open heart and mind and really consider why you picked up this book and what you want to do to change your life...because it WILL change your life.

Ok, back to my story, I struggled with my weight when I was in middle school and high school. I may not have been perceived as being overweight, but I wasn't comfortable in my own skin, and I struggled to eat right. I thought working out gave me the permission to keep eating poorly, and I truly had no concept of what it took to control my weight. After high school, I tried to eat better, and I exercised A LOT, but even though I lost weight and felt better, I still had only found a temporary solution. Then, it was time to go off to college...and guess what?! I put on, yes, the dreaded freshman 15! I wasn't necessarily eating poorly...but we will dive more into that topic later. Then, I was home for the summer between my freshman and sophomore years, and I decided to start running, which I continued into my sophomore year with some friends...but then certain life circumstances kept me from continuing. So, fast-forward to the summer between my sophomore and junior year, I started running again, AND I added in biking. A good friend and I literally biked around 30 miles every couple of days. I was in the best-shape of my life after that summer! Can you guess what's coming next? Yep, a big emotional life event! Life sure can be a roller coaster at times, can't it?! Well, needless to say, the next several years involved a lot of ups and downs...both with emotions and weight gain/loss.

I hope this gives you a decent picture of my background...and how my journey began. I'm thankful that this is all in the past, and that I am moving forward with my life. How about you? Are you ready to ditch the junk and move forward...and find your spunk? Who wants to be stuck in a funk? Not me!!! My first "aha" moment was when I read a book by Gwen Shamblin called *The Weigh Down Diet*. It's been several years since I read the book, but my biggest take away was to not let food have an emotional pull on you and to stop eating when you are full...and not eating again until you are hungry. This way of thinking helped me a lot, but after having my thyroid removed, I realized I needed something more. You wouldn't believe the amount of time I have spent researching and searching for answers! I've had a desire in my heart since I was 18 years old to help myself and others be free from weight struggles. Those struggling with thyroid issues know that even when you think you are doing everything right, the scale won't budge...and sometimes keeps creeping up. Hence my desire to find answers.

This brings me to the last leg of my journey...life without a thyroid. When I first had my thyroid removed (followed by radioactive iodine to kill all the remaining thyroid cells in my body), my doctors put me on Synthroid and suppressed my TSH levels for several years because they said this would keep any thyroid cells from growing back. I did okay with my weight and energy for a while, but after a certain point my medicine didn't seem to be working (despite a low TSH). Not only did I start getting hives from the medication, but I also felt tired all of the time and started to have issues with weight again, along with several other typical hypothyroid symptoms. So, being the researcher that I am, I decided to start reading books and online articles about metabolism. At the time, I was doing several of Jillian Michael's workout programs and I decided to purchase her *Master Your Metabolism* book. I learned that she had thyroid issues too, and she explained about the active thyroid hormone (T3), which then lead me on a quest to learn more about the different thyroid hormones. For about ten years, I trusted that the TSH lab test was the way to measure your thyroid levels, but soon learned that it was technically a pituitary hormone level, and that it doesn't necessarily reflect how well your thyroid (or thyroid medication) is performing. Therefore, armed with this new information, I decided to ask my Endocrinologist if he would check my Free T3 levels...and his response, "That's an expensive test, and I wouldn't treat you any differently." As a result, that was my last visit with that doctor. This was around the same time that I discovered Facebook support groups as well as individuals like Gena Lee Nolin (*Thyroid Sexy* on Facebook) and additional thyroid supports like *Stop The Thyroid Madness*. They helped open my eyes to see that it was more than just the TSH lab test results, and I had the right to fire my doctor and find someone who would help me to find optimal thyroid levels.

I should mention that during the last couple of years trying to figure things out with my thyroid levels, etc., I was actually dealing with nerve issues. It started with a little tingling and numbness in my right hand (which I first thought was a trapped nerve). However, I eventually started to feel the tingling/numbness in my right foot (peripheral neuropathy) as well. So, I made an appointment to see one of the physicians in the doctor's group where I belong and during my visit I told the doctor that I thought I was starting to feel it on the left side, too. Well, it eventually spread throughout my body (with accompanying pain in the back of my legs) and even to the top of my head. The night that I felt it in my head is still a very vivid memory. My parents had arrived earlier that day because we were getting ready to go on our yearly trip to Hilton Head, and everyone was settling for bed so that we could leave early in the morning. Right before getting in bed, I told my husband, Greg, that I thought I was starting to feel the nerve stuff on the top of my head. I had already been feeling it in my back, but this was a new feeling for me. So, I made myself relax and go to sleep. I had only been asleep for about an hour when I woke up because it felt like the nerves were doing a wave through my body...from head to toe! So, I woke my hubby up and told him that he needed to take me to the emergency room...because I was freaked out by what was happening. I also woke my mom up to tell her that we were headed to the emergency room, and she would have to listen for our boys. By the time we arrived at the emergency room, the waves had stopped, but I still had them check me out to make sure I was okay to travel. They never found anything and released me to go on vacation, and told me to check in with my primary care doctor when I arrived back home. After the fact, it's funny to hear my husband retell the story because he said they thought I was on drugs...because they were asking me the same questions as they were asking the person in the room next to me who was there due to actually overdosing on drugs. It was a scary time in my life because I had no idea what was going on with me, and I had extreme pain in the back of my legs that made it hurt to sit or stand for any length of time. Consequently, this pain and numbness was what kept me searching for answers when all the doctors (2 Internal Medicine, 2 Neurologist, 2 Endocrinologist, and one Specialist) couldn't figure out what was wrong with me.

Additional issues that I've endured along the way have played a role in helping me discover the keys to unlocking the door to optimal wellness. On top of the hypothyroid symptoms and nerve issues that I have previously mentioned, I've also dealt with Raynaud's, two frozen shoulders (and coinciding inflammation), major life stressors, discovering food intolerances, perimenopause, Epstein Barre Virus, Candida, Small Intestinal Bacterial Overgrowth (SIBO), and leaky gut. So, I'm no stranger to pain and discomfort. However, it's my hope and prayer that my struggles can help you discover your optimal wellness as you learn to ditch the junk and find your spunk! Are you ready? I hope so...let's go!

Chapter 1

DO Take Care of YOU!

I want to start by saying that I'm not typically a fan of stating the negative by telling people what NOT to do; however, besides the catchy title, this book will walk you through the process of letting go of those things that are holding all of us back from an abundant, most-optimal life. Just like a tree must be pruned to bear good fruit, we too need to go through a pruning process to be our best selves. So, I would encourage you to read the chapters with an open heart and mind and think of this process as a part of pruning away the yuck to allow for the positive to grow. Ask yourself, "Do I want to find optimal wellness, or do I want to continue living and feeling the way I do now?" Are you ready to take care of you?

My number one piece of advice I always tell others is, Be Your Own Advocate! You have to take the lead on your health! There is NO ONE who knows your body better than you, and if you think that something seems off, you're most likely correct. If you've been told your thyroid labs are "normal," but you're still having symptoms, don't just settle. The same goes for any issues you're having with your health. Action is required if you want to see change! Therefore, you may need to search for a new doctor, make changes to your diet or daily habits, or look into a different treatment approach/plan.

• • •

FIND YOUR SPUNK TIP:
Be Your Own Advocate ~ Find Root Cause
(Don't Treat Symptoms)

• • •

My hope is to arm you with the right tools so that you have the confidence to fight for your health...and sometimes it's just having the wisdom to make certain changes on your own (things that don't require medical intervention, like eating healthier). One of the best things you can do for yourself is to search for the root cause of the symptoms you are dealing with, not just treating symptoms. When you treat symptoms, it just becomes a vicious cycle, and you will have a difficult time moving forward with your health. Treating symptoms only provides instant gratification, but it will not get you the end results you desire. If you want optimal wellness, it is crucial to find the root of the issue. Otherwise, it will be like those stubborn nettle weeds, you think you have gotten rid of them, but if you didn't get the whole root they will come back...and worse than the first time. Go for the root!!!

When you find me on social media, you will see that I love to share thyroid tips...and I even have a special day that I focus on thyroid-related information (e.g., Thyroid Thursday). Fortunately, I like to research because after having lived without a thyroid for over sixteen years I have encountered a number of issues that I have had to face. When you consider that every cell in our body needs thyroid hormone to function properly, it is apparent, in fact, essential that we need to maintain optimal thyroid levels. If we have decreased thyroid functioning, we will face a myriad of symptoms that will affect our quality of life. However, this book is more than just about our thyroids...although that is a key player, it is more about discovering the key principles for finding optimal wellness (in EVERY area of our lives). Consequently, I'll be sharing key thyroid steps that I have taken to find my optimal levels/wellness, but I will also share other health tips and the plan I used and continue to use to stay healthy and find optimal wellness.

Chapter 2

Ditch the TSH Only Lab Testing

What is TSH and why am I addressing this topic early on in my book? First, I mentioned TSH in my introduction, but if you are reading this book and you are not aware of what TSH means, or what the results of the TSH lab test marker means, let me give you a quick explanation. TSH stands for Thyroid-Stimulating Hormone, and it is produced by the pituitary gland. The pituitary gland, which sits at the base of the brain, receives orders from the hypothalamus, and it's the main control of hormone production in our bodies. One of its primary jobs is to stimulate the thyroid gland to produce thyroxine (also known as T4) and smaller amounts of triiodothyronin (T3) (about 20% compared to 80% of the T4 production). Essentially, the TSH lab measures how much T4 the pituitary gland is asking the thyroid gland to make. T3 is the active thyroid hormone, and if our bodies are functioning optimally then T4 will convert into T3 when needed. The issue arises when our bodies aren't doing a good job of converting the T4 into T3.

Our thyroid gland is the key regulator of our metabolism. So, if we are not producing adequate amounts of thyroid hormone or our bodies are not converting well, then we will most likely end up in a hypothyroid state. When our thyroid levels are not optimal, our metabolism will be more sluggish and we will face many of the typical hypothyroid symptoms. Unfortunately, when one hormone is off, it tends to have an effect on the other hormones. For instance, thyroid functioning may decrease when cortisol levels are out of control due to the impact it has on our adrenals. It's kind of like a Domino effect, and we could experience a whole array of hormone issues involving imbalances with the thyroid and other hormones like estrogen, progesterone, and testosterone.

Secondly, I wanted to address this topic early on in my book because I believe there are far more people (especially women) who are suffering from thyroid imbalances than are being identified. When we look solely to the TSH lab marker, we can miss a key factor in how our thyroid is functioning. As I mentioned above, T3 is our active thyroid hormone, and for those people who are not good T4-to-T3 converters, the TSH result doesn't give an accurate picture of what is actually going on. So, when I say "Ditch the TSH Lab Only Testing," I'm suggesting we don't rely solely on this marker when evaluating true thyroid functioning. I'm not against the TSH lab marker because it does have its place. However, I believe it's just a piece of the puzzle, and we need to put all the pieces together to solve the whole puzzle and find our true answer. For example, even when my various doctors were suppressing my TSH because they didn't want my thyroid cells to grow back, I still experienced hypothyroid symptoms. I was constantly told that my labs were "normal" and it was just the fact that I was getting older. Well, if you know anything about me, you most likely know that I am not one to just accept an answer like that (and you shouldn't either)...because I know that growing older does not doom you to growing bigger! So, as I mentioned in the intro, this is what propelled me into my search for how to increase my metabolism and how I learned about the other thyroid markers. Therefore, I would encourage you to also look beyond the TSH when you're searching for answers.

Before we move on, I want to make sure you realize the significant consequences our thyroid functioning has on our health. The breadth of the impact on all of our other body systems and functions is the bigger issue. My hope is that once you see the impact it has on our overall health, you will realize why I'm so passionate about teaching others about taking care of your thyroid AND making sure you ask for a full thyroid panel (not just the TSH marker) when looking for answers to health questions. We will talk more on balancing our thyroid hormones in a future chapter, but I want you to take a look at some of the ways thyroid disease can affect our health. According to Mary Shomon, author of *The Thyroid Menopause Solution*, thyroid problems not only play a role in slowing down the metabolism (and weight loss resistance...due to unstable blood sugar), but they can have an impact during our perimenopausal/menopausal years as well. Not only are we at risk for starting menopause earlier, but we run the risk of having worsening symptoms. Plus, one of the symptoms that Shomon listed is one that frustrates me when I hear that someone is not receiving proper thyroid care, and that is the fact that a slow thyroid can impair our effectiveness to deal with illnesses or recovery. Guys and gals...our immune system needs optimal thyroid functioning to protect and heal us!!! Our thyroid functioning impacts many different body systems. I'm guessing you may know someone who has had either a thyroid nodule(s) or a goiter (enlarged thyroid); however, did you know that our thyroid functioning can have an impact on our cholesterol, blood pressure, triglyceride levels, and heart health? Regarding heart health, if you do a web search on low T3 levels and heart failure, you will most likely find several studies showing a link between the two. I found several in my search. For example, one study published in *The American Journal of Medicine* found an improvement in cardiac function by increasing T3 hormone levels. Likewise, another one published by *ESC Heart Fail*, which was a double-blind, placebo controlled study, showed multiple benefits for the patients who were in the synthetic T3 therapy group.

There are many other conditions that are fairly common in people with Hashimoto's and hypothyroidism besides those listed, so be aware that symptoms you may be experiencing could also be linked to your thyroid levels. In fact, when I found out that my blood results indicated I had Candida and that I had evidence of having the Epstein Barre virus in the past, one of my doctors indicated that it is frequently seen in those who have Hashimoto's. So, regardless of root cause, there is a high correlation between these conditions. Interestingly, whenever I have experienced any of the commonly linked conditions (including Plantar fasciitis and potentially fibromyalgia), my symptoms have always improved when my thyroid levels have been optimized. Therefore, regardless of initial cause, I have noticed optimal thyroid levels make a significant difference in my overall health.

Well...have I convinced you of the importance of requesting a full thyroid panel yet?

• • •

FIND YOUR SPUNK TIP:
Request a Full Thyroid Panel & Corresponding Labs

• • •

As a result of my experience and everything that I have learned along the way, I have discovered that it is important to request a full thyroid panel (and corresponding labs). After many years of being told my thyroid levels were "normal" based off of the TSH lab along with learning that T3 is your active thyroid hormone, I decided to find someone who would check all the involved labs. As suspected, despite having a "normal" TSH, my T3 levels were in the "hypo" range...and since T3 is the active thyroid hormone, I was having hypothyroid symptoms despite "normal" labs. Therefore, I believe it's important to include labs such as Free T4, Free T3, Reverse T3, TPO (Thyroid Peroxidase Antibodies), and TSI (Thyroid Stimulating Immunoglobulin) to get a better picture of what is happening in our bodies. In addition, if we are deficient in certain vitamins or minerals it can have an impact on our thyroid levels. So, it's important to check these corresponding labs as well to make sure everything is within the normal range (e.g., iron, B12, Vitamin D). The key is to look at the big picture. If we look at only one lab marker then we could be missing important pieces of the puzzle to get to the root cause of our issues.

Personally, after all of my research (and a lot of prayer and consulting), I decided that I wanted to find a doctor that was willing to run a complete lab panel of tests and who would let me try natural thyroid medication (instead of the synthetic). It wasn't easy finding someone, and there have been some bumps along the way. However, after finding a new doctor who helped me to work towards finding my optimal thyroid levels, the switch has been life-changing! It was truly amazing the difference I felt and how much energy I gained. The time that I became more aware of the difference was on a family vacation in Hilton Head. For many years, we would go to Hilton Head, and every afternoon I would send my family off to do something fun while I went to take an afternoon nap. The year that I switched to WP Thyroid [a name brand for a natural dessicated thyroid medication (NDT)], my family mentioned about going off to do something in the afternoon, and I was eager to join in on the fun. So, when I say it was life-changing, I truly mean that it was LIFE-CHANGING! I cannot imagine ever having to go back to the life that I thought I was destined to...of low energy and never feeling up to doing all the cool stuff with my family and friends. Making the switch was the best decision, for my health, I ever made!

If you would like to know more about what I've learned on my thyroid journey, and key experts whom I follow, I've included information and links in the appendix section. I've also included information and references regarding recommended labs, optimal levels, and additional labs or supplements that are good for those with decreased thyroid functioning (or no thyroid). Plus, within this book you will find information on how all of the hormones can affect each other as well as keys to balancing all of our hormones. Lastly, I want to provide you with my key resources that I've used for optimal thyroid health. I believe making these changes will help you find your spunk, too.

Chapter 3

Ditch the Endocrine Disruptors

Wait, what is an endocrine disruptor? An endocrine disruptor or an endocrine-disrupting chemical (EDC) as defined by The Endocrine Society (Gore, et al.) as, "an exogenous [non-natural] chemical, or mixture of chemicals, that interferes with any aspect of hormone action." More simply, it's a chemical that throws off your hormones (e.g., thyroid, estrogen, progesterone). They are said to either mimic or block a natural hormone.

The Endocrine Society has put together a great resource to provide us with information about endocrine disrupting chemicals. The following resource: *Introduction to Endocrine Disrupting Chemicals (EDCs): A Guide for Public Interest*

Organizations and Policy-Makers can be found in the reference section. They noted, "Because of the endocrine system's critical role in so many important biological and physiological functions, impairments in any part of the endocrine system can lead to disease or even death. By interfering with the body's endocrine systems, EDC exposure can therefore perturb many functions." They further explain how it has become a global problem because of the many places from which we are exposed, including the air we breathe and by ingesting certain foods and drinks. We can also come into contact with them through our skin, and they can be transferred in vitro (from mother to fetus) as well as through breast milk. They suggested there could be around 1,000 manufactured chemicals that may have endocrine-acting properties.

Additionally, what many don't realize is that these chemicals build up in our systems over time (bioaccumulate), and we can have what is referred to as body burden, which is the amount of endocrine disruptors that we have accumulated over the years. In fact, the Endocrine Society stated that nearly 100% of humans have a body burden as measured by biomonitoring techniques that show detectable levels of chemicals in our blood, urine, placenta, and umbilical cord blood. Therefore, the issue arises when we assume that we have not been affected by the chemicals because we do not have an immediate response. Unfortunately, the real test will most likely be years down the road when our bodies start to feel the effects and most probably will not realize the cause/connection. It's impossible to totally eliminate our exposure to endocrine disruptors, but we can take charge of what is in our control and start making changes today.

My introduction to endocrine disruptors began with my diagnosis of thyroid cancer. I wasn't diagnosed with the most typical type of thyroid cancer, so I wanted to learn more about the type that I was diagnosed with...and learn what caused it. During my research, I discovered that they were not really sure of the cause of Follicular Cell Thyroid Cancer, but it was thought to be linked to pesticides. So, that is when I started trying to remove pesticides in my foods...which was a slow process. However, it wasn't until a few years ago that I discovered that there were endocrine disruptors EVERYWHERE!!! They lurk in our foods, the soil, our water, personal care products, our household cleaners, our makeup, medicines, air fresheners, candles, plastics, store receipts...and the list goes on! I honestly had no idea! That's why I believe knowledge is power. I didn't know, and you might not know, the dangers that are lurking within the walls of your home. It saddens me that we let these chemicals into our homes and expose ourselves and our children to them unknowingly. Had I previously known this information, I never would have used any of these products. My hope is to educate you, so that you can have the knowledge and power to ditch these dangers before they cause further harm to you or your family members.

I am encouraged to see that an increasing number of people are becoming aware of certain ingredients that are found in our everyday beauty or skin-care products that can be disruptive to our hormones and thyroid functioning. One of the first endocrine disruptors that I learned about was the chemical paraben, which is added to many of our beauty products (shampoos, lotions, soaps, shaving gel, toothpaste, cosmetics). I've even seen it listed in certain common over-the-counter medicines. It's considered a synthetic estrogen, and it's used as a preservative in many personal care products (including children's) and some are allowed in foods. This chemical has many different names, so, it's important to check out the ingredient lists and avoid products if you see any of the following: butyl-, ethyl-, methyl-, or propylparaben. The good news is that it's becoming easier to find paraben-free products.

Before I continue, let me state that there are several other known endocrine disrupting chemicals, which I will briefly share in this chapter to help explain why it's important to ditch products that we use that contain them. I will also provide additional links in the appendix section on where you can find more detail/information on endocrine disprutors. I want you to see the need to be mindful of these ingredients, but I also don't want to overwhelm anyone with details. So, feel free to flip to the back of the book to learn where you can go to get more information on endocrine disrupting chemicals.

This next one was a surprise to me since it's a commonly used ingredient that's touted as being good for you. Any guesses??? It's fluoride...and it's definitely not a friend to our thyroids. Did you know that in the past, fluoride was used to treat an overactive thyroid? Yikes! In fact, the following Stop The Thyroid Madness post: *Fluoride and your Thyroid-a dangerous connection.*, indicated that "fluoride compounds were added to the drinking water of prisoners to keep them docile and inhibit questioning of authority, both in Nazi prison camps in World War II and in the Soviet gulags in Siberia." Kind of scary, isn't it?! This link is also provided in the appendix if you want more details. This just goes to show that endocrine disruptors can be hidden in unlikely places. Therefore, we need to arm ourselves with information that will help us make empowered decisions.

Endocrine Disruptors are literally EVERYWHERE!!! Places you might expect to find them include gasoline and pesticides (including glyphosate...which has been found in the foods we eat, too), but they are also in common household cleaners, plastic food containers and wraps (including medical tubing), electronics and building materials, personal care products, stain resistant carpet, furniture, and clothing, non-stick pans, and antibacterial products. Even children's products have been found to contain EDC's like lead, phthalates, and cadmium. Also, sometimes the endocrine disruptor is not indicated on the product. For example, it might just say, "added fragrance." This typically means it contains phthalates. Lastly, we have to watch for it in our food (e.g., pesticides, phytoestrogens, and mercury) and water (e.g., fluoride, chlorine, and heavy metals). This is not an exhaustive list, but it should give you a good idea of how widespread endocrine disruptors are in our environment. In addition, for my thyroid peeps...and/or those who are in the 40 years of age and older crowd like me, I would highly recommend Mary Shomon's book, *The Menopause Thyroid Solution*. She has a lot of helpful information, but she also goes more in depth about all the endocrine disruptors and other exposures that can cause or increase our chances of thyroid issues. These include: autoimmune thyroid conditions and hypothyroidism.

Oh, and did you know that these chemicals can have an impact on your weight? Yep, according to the Endocrine Society, "Chemicals referred to as "obesogens" are thought to enhance weight gain by altering or reprogramming key parts of the endocrine system governing metabolism, energy balance, and appetite, resulting in obesity and its related adverse health outcomes." These chemicals can disrupt thyroid hormone function, affecting our metabolisms, which is why I decided long ago to ditch the endocrine disruptors. Who wants to use/ingest chemicals that could make you gain weight? Not me!!!

• • •

FIND YOUR SPUNK TIP:
Choose Chemical-Free Whenever Possible

• • •

What can we do to reduce our exposure? It's time to ditch and switch! With food, we need to aim for minimal ingredients and real food and to choose organic whenever possible. Plus, we need to get rid of any personal care or household product that can interfere with your endocrine system. Balancing hormones can be hard enough on its own, but when we mix in endocrine disruptors our bodies go haywire. In a world where it seems like so many things are out of our control, THIS is something that we can control. However, only you can make that decision. The quicker we make these changes, the better! We want to reduce the bioaccumulation and body burden that is created by using these endocrine disrupting chemicals. This moves us one step closer to finding our spunk! Woohoo!

Chapter 4

Ditch Food Intolerances & Antinutrients

Now, let's talk about food and how it plays a role in our thyroid and overall health. If you are like most people (myself included) who I encounter, food choices can be a sensitive topic; however, I believe it's a key component to finding our optimal. I believe Hippocrates nailed it on the head when he said, "Let food be thy medicine and medicine be thy food." Although many are unaware, many of us have dealt with and/or are dealing with food intolerances. The sensitivity often stems from an underlying issue with the health of our gut. In fact, my doctor refers to food intolerances as "messengers." In the case of food intolerances, the message is that there is a breakdown in the gastrointestinal tract (GI) tract.

Regardless, it is an issue that we need to face. Gluten and dairy intolerances seem to be common with those with autoimmune thyroid disease. In fact, I knew that dairy caused me issues on occasion, but I never really understood the impact it was having on my body. Food intolerances set off a chain reaction, which begins by gradually causing inflammatory antibodies to build up in the intestines, but it may also travel to the skin and joints. Also, when the liver becomes inflamed from the food intolerances, the chain reaction causes a drop in blood sugar levels, leading to food cravings. Before I discovered that I had a gut issue, I remember wondering, "Why am I craving chips or corn chips so much?!" To top it all off, if we have a fungal overgrowth like Candida (which, I did), the foods we are craving are most likely ones that feed the fungal overgrowth. Urg! Consequently, these food intolerances can have a negative impact on our gut bacteria. Plus, with all of this internal stress, we may experience the negative effects of cortisol too, because it's a huge contributor in the roller coaster ride of chain reactions...but we will talk more about that later. Many of the symptoms of food intolerance that I experienced include:

- Constipation
- Bloating

- Rashes/Hives
- Fatigue
- Stuffy nose or post nasal drip
- Brain fog and difficulty concentrating
- Joint pain
- Cravings
- Weight gain (but some may experience weight loss)

However, our son also experienced some behavior issues when dealing with food intolerance...and his behavior improved after removing the offending foods from his diet. Additionally, others might experience symptoms such as acid reflux, headaches, stomach aches, or eczema.

Did you know that bloating is not a normal occurrence? I never really thought about it until I realized I had true food intolerances when I was trying to figure out why I was having inflammation pain in my legs. I decided to do a cleanse which phased out gluten and dairy (among a few other foods), and by the end I had a significant decrease in the inflammation. Plus, after realizing these two foods were the main culprits, I continued to omit them from my diet, and the inflammation pain eventually went away. I had moments at the beginning when I would sneak bites of these foods, but I would notice the inflammation returning. So, it became a no-brainer for me to eliminate them from my diet. I basically had to weigh the choices, do I want to feel good or do I want to enjoy a bite of the offending food (which would be gone in no time)? I decided the momentary pleasure wasn't worth the pain that it caused.

I mentioned that gluten and dairy seem to be common food sensitivities for those with an autoimmune thyroid disease; however, I should also add that it is highly recommended that this same population avoid gluten due to the effect it can have on the thyroid. According to Dr. Myers, "every time they [those with autoimmune thyroid disease] eat gluten the immune system sends out antibodies to detect and destroy the gluten, but since the gluten and thyroid gland looks so similar, some of those immune cells end up attacking the thyroid by mistake." Consequently, I would highly encourage you to consider this impact on your thyroid before you consume any more gluten. (Note: The gluten we eat today is not the same gluten that our grandparents/great-grandparents ate. It has been modified greatly.)

Do you know if you have any food intolerances? There are food sensitivity tests, many of which can be fairly costly. However, if you don't want to pay for testing, you can also go through a process of eliminating foods and then re-adding them one at a time back into your diet, noting any changes that occur. Several years ago I participated in a three-week non-fasting cleanse that helped to reveal sensitivities that I had to gluten and dairy. However, more recently, after dealing with hives my Integrative Medicine doctor put in a lab request in order to check my IgG (immunoglobulin G) reactions to the top six allergens. This lab test does not test for true allergies, instead it looks for foods that cause a delayed reaction. Aside from one test the lab did in error (peanuts), my results indicated that I had a positive reaction to the remaining six items: oats, corn, wheat, dairy, eggs, and soy. So, these are definitely items that I would urge you to consider ditching for a time to see if you notice a difference when they are reintroduced.

Interestingly, during my research on an anti-Candida diet I came across information from JJ Virgin, CNS, CHFS, an internationally recognized fitness, nutrition, and weight-loss expert, on the most common food intolerances she encountered. Her list was similar, but did not include the oats (and it had the addition of sugar on her list). Although sugar is not a true food "intolerance," I would agree that it's good for EVERYONE to ditch the sugar. Cutting sugar, and foods that turn to sugar has made a big impact in helping my body to heal. Sugar essentially feeds the bad bacteria in our guts (which we will discuss more later), and it works against our healing process. So, as far as the foods that we have discussed as potential offenders, it might be good to test them all. Oats were actually my highest reaction, and our youngest son has an intolerance to it as well, so it would definitely be on my recommended list. The eight items would include:

- Peanuts
- Oats
- Corn
- Gluten
- Dairy
- Soy
- Sugar
- Eggs

Removing food intolerances is only the start of the process, but you would be amazed at the changes you will most likely experience when removing these foods. Just think about all of the internal inflammation it must cause in our bodies. I cannot even imagine! I know the hives were miserable!!! When I removed these eight items from my diet, my hives went away...and my energy increased greatly. Plus, I finally started to notice a difference in the scale. I believe this shows us the significant effect that food intolerances have on our bodies...and why we should be mindful of them. I learned the hard way, but my hope is to teach others so they can learn from my experience.

Let me back up a little and start with the beginning of my journey, which began over 16 years ago when I learned that soy could have a negative impact on our thyroid functioning. I decided to remove it from my diet. Then, a few years ago I removed gluten and dairy after realizing my body was much happier without it. I try to eat only natural sugars and started removing peanuts/peanut butter from my diet about a year ago. So, from the list above I had essentially removed everything but corn, eggs, and oats...and a little natural sugar. However, I had started noticing some issues when I would eat corn chips so I decided to take a break from them. Consequently, I later discovered I had Candida, which can cause our bodies to become sensitive to more foods, and it causes you to crave foods you shouldn't eat. Unfortunately, corn chips are one of the foods that Candida thrives on (and I later discovered it was a food I had become sensitive to). So, I am thankful that I had already chosen to remove it from my diet. Was it easy...NO! Was it worth it? YES!!! Anyone who knows me well, knows that I love corn chips, but I had to make a choice. However, I can tell you that I am very happy with my decision. Therefore, if you want to feel optimal, this is a critical piece to the puzzle!

By the way, if you are not familiar with how to do an elimination diet and are looking for a specific elimination diet protocol to follow, I will make sure to provide suggested resources on where to find this information. However, the basic gist of an elimination diet is to start by eliminating the potential food intolerances, and then one-by-one adding them back in to see if any of them cause you issues. If certain foods do not cause you any issues, then you can keep them in your diet. However, if you notice ANY type of symptoms, then these foods need to be ditched for a time until your gut has healed. Since food intolerances wreak havoc on our guts and put our immune system on high alert, our bodies tend to overreact to the foods we eat. So, we must begin by letting our immune system "chill out" before re-introducing potential food intolerances back into our diets.

Now, let's address antinutrients since they often display similar issues as seen with food intolerances (e.g., gut and autoimmune reactions). It's amazing the things you learn when you are searching for answers! Believe it or not, many antinutrients are found in foods that we consider to be healthy, like beans, seeds, and raw cruciferous veggies (e.g., broccoli, cauliflower, cabbage, kale, Brussels sprouts). Crazy, isn't it?! Some of the key antinutrients are lectins, oxalates, phytates, and mold toxins. I'm not going to dive too deep into this area because it's something that can be easily found in a web search, but I think it's important to note that antinutrients can cause issues with proper mineral and nutrient absorption (robbing our bodies of the nutrients when we eat them) due to the effect they have on our digestive enzymes.

Therefore, individuals, who have a sensitivity, need to be mindful of how their body reacts when they eat certain foods, remembering these antinutrients can be found in healthy foods (as noted above). One particular antinutrient, oxalates, drew my attention because the consumption of oxalates has been found to be an issue for individuals that deal with kidney stones on a regular basis. Sadly enough, since oxalates are found in healthy foods, most individuals who eat a high oxalate diet are typically people who are healthier eaters. So, don't discount this chapter just because you are a "healthy" eater. I believe we all should pay attention to how our body reacts to the foods that we choose to eat.

I should also mention goitrogenic foods since they are foods that can interfere with proper thyroid hormone production. These foods can prevent the body from using iodine when making thyroid hormone and in turn may cause the formation of goiters (enlargement of thyroid) and/or hypothyroidism. I do have to say that this is probably the only positive aspect about not having a thyroid...because I don't have to worry about goitrogens since it only applies to those who still have a functional thyroid gland. However, for those of you who still have a functional thyroid, I would caution against eating too many goitrogens. Goitrogen foods include raw cruciferous vegetables and soy products. Cruciferous vegetables have a reduced effect if they are cooked, and most potent when they are consumed raw. So, rather than eliminating these foods that are rich in key nutrients, it would be wiser to limit eating raw cruciferous vegetables and opt for the cooked version. In addition, organic and fermented soy (e.g., Natto, Miso) seem to be less of a concern, and, therefore, a better choice. If you want to regain your spunk, you must take care of your thyroid!

Okay, dare I mention it? Caffeine...some people seem to tolerate it well, but others do not. So, before we move on, let's touch on coffee since it is a staple in the diet of many. Is it healthy, or not? There seems to be a debate going on, and there is research to show some of the benefits; however, I know from personal experience that certain populations need to be careful about their caffeine intake. For example, I was told at the age of 18 that I should avoid caffeine due to fibrocystic disease. Plus, reducing or eliminating caffeine is also recommended for those with thyroid disease due to the increased demand on the adrenal glands. Caffeine spikes our cortisol, and if we are having issues with our adrenal function, then it could place an extra burden on our adrenals. As a result, anyone who is under a lot of stress (external or internal) should be mindful of consuming too much caffeine. This would include anyone who is dealing with a variety of different health issues. Therefore, we must consider our individual situations and determine if the benefits outweigh the consequences.

I do want to note that in my research I also discovered another important aspect to consider with coffee. There apparently is a large percentage of coffee on the market today that is not clean. This does not include all the unhealthy ingredients that people add in...including a large amount of sugar. A fairly small percentage of coffee is organically grown, which means you're most likely drinking coffee that is filled with pesticides. So, if you are a coffee fan (and not sensitive to the caffeine), then it would be wise to choose a brand that is clean, and preferably organic. It's better to be safe than sorry!

Lastly, I want to mention a couple of tidbits I learned about alcohol. When we drink alcohol it turns into acetaldehyde when it is broken down in our livers...which creates an internal toxic environment. Also, interesting to note, did you know that alcohol messes with estrogen levels??? Like coffee, there has been evidence for positive and negative effects; however, as with all of the nutrients we eat or drink we must pay attention to our own individual reactions. What proves to be a non-issue for one person may be a huge issue for another. For this reason, we must be our own health advocates, because we are not all cut from the same cookie cutter. All of what I am sharing in this book is about helping you to learn how to listen to your own body and not depend on what everyone else is doing. If you listen long enough and hard enough, your body will tell you what it needs, or what it should go without.

• • •

FIND YOUR SPUNK TIP:
Keep a Food Journal & Add Healing Foods

• • •

The cool part in all of this is that by removing food intolerances and/or antinutrients, it typically results in a double blessing! Number one, you feel better...physically, mentally, and emotionally. Who doesn't want to feel better??? Blessing number two, weight loss! Hello, you mean I don't have to reduce my calories, just remove my food intolerances or the typical food sensitivities and I will lose weight? I have heard it said that inflammation is the biggest cause of "muffin top," and it's probably true. Once we ditch the foods that are causing inflammation in our guts then we can begin our journey to healing and wellness. The key is to learn tasty swaps for the foods that you are removing and making sure you are eating the right kinds of food to support your digestion and metabolism.

In regards to antinutrients, it's not always necessary to remove these foods from our diet (unless we are sensitive), but we can make necessary changes in how we prepare these foods. For instance, I've started soaking my chia seeds and flaxseeds, and I switched to sprouted flaxseeds. In addition, I am now eating more fermented vegetables. I have been gradually adding them into my diet. When you soak, sprout, or ferment seeds it makes them easier to digest. I should add that this includes nuts, beans, legumes, and grain seeds. Steaming or cooking high oxalate foods and cruciferous veggies can help reduce the negative effects as well. Oh, and a cool piece of info that I learned from Donna Gates, the author of *Body Ecology*, is that fermenting vegetables can add an extra benefit. She explained that the microbiota found in fermented vegetables will help eat up the garbage...or "poisons" that we eat. Therefore, it seems preparation of antinutrient foods is the key, we can reduce the negative properties by soaking and sprouting seeds, steaming/cooking, and fermenting veggies.

Additionally, since I painted more of a negative picture about coffee above, I should note an interesting fact I learned about coffee. Coffee is full of antioxidants and polyphenols, so it's not all bad. Plus, there is research that shows that coffee helps to heal the liver (Ratini 2017)...and we know that caffeine can help boost our metabolism and therefore increase our work effort during our exercise sessions. So, provided our adrenal glands are healthy, and we are not under extra stress (internal or external), then drinking a cup or two of clean coffee appears to be beneficial. The key is to know what works best for you and know when to take a break when needed. If energy is the reason you choose to drink coffee, we will talk more on that in a bit.

On a personal note, at the time of writing this book, I'm still in the testing phase of figuring out the exact cause of my food intolerances, which is most likely due to a leaky gut and potential SIBO. Plus, I want to make sure I am not sensitive to any antinutrients. I have had occasional histamine reactions after eating certain foods, which I now know are related to a particular food intolerance that I didn't know I had. However, the bigger issue is determining what is at the root of the issue and how I can work to eliminate the intolerances (and eventually add some foods back into my diet). I'm glad I went ahead and did the blood testing to check for the big seven food intolerances because I have seen the positive effects it had on our youngest son by identifying and removing the offenders.

Our son actually had more extensive testing done and it was interesting to learn about the foods that were triggers for him. We were surprised by some of the foods listed. His list included items such as gluten, peanuts, egg yolks, and a couple dairy products; however, he also had sensitivities to healthier foods such as olive oil, oats, and flaxseed. Therefore, keep in mind that the above list is only the most frequently seen food intolerances, it's not an exhaustive list. It is, however, a good place to start.

Planning, tracking, and journaling are important for anyone trying to make changes in his/her health and diet. One of the biggest keys to eliminating food intolerances or figuring out if you have any sensitivities to any foods is meal planning. Without the proper planning, we are left to scrounge on what is readily available to us. I would also encourage you to use a food journal to keep track of your symptoms and record if anything changes or if symptoms seem to be worse at one time versus another. When you have a record it allows you to compare your symptoms to see if anything shows a connection. This helps us to better express our symptoms to our health care provider. Plus, many times with food intolerances (since they are not true allergies), it may take a couple of days before we see a reaction from the offending food. By journaling, we become more aware of how we are feeling, and it helps us to become more in tune with our bodies. In general, food journaling helps us to be more mindful of what we are consuming.

Lastly, I want to make sure to note that most food intolerances are temporary, and many people can return to eating most of these foods once you have discovered the source of the issues and cleaned up your gut. However, I am personally not a fan of soy, and I'd rather avoid it because a large percentage of soy is genetically modified (as is corn). Plus, many believe soy is not friendly to the thyroid or to optimal thyroid functioning. Next, most of the gluten you find on the market today is not the real deal...so I would use caution and urge you not to go hog wild with this nutrient. Overall, even if you do reintroduce some of these foods and do not experience any immediate negative effects, these are foods that are best kept to a minimum in your diet. Therefore, until we go through the process of eliminating offending foods, we will always be shooting in the dark and wondering what is causing the issues we are facing. So, I would encourage you to consider ditching these common food intolerances to clean up your gut and help reset your body to burn food more efficiently.

Chapter 5

Ditch One Size Fits All Diets

There are tons of different diets or eating plans being promoted, and I am sure you've seen ads trying to tell you that THIS is the best one for you. Well, as a certified Health Coach, I can explain the different options and show you what research shows as far as results. However, I cannot design a specific eating plan for you. One thing I know for sure is that there is not a one size fits all diet. I believe there are some general rules that apply to all; however, we are all unique with different genes and different health needs (e.g., diabetic, thyroid disease, adrenal fatigue, SIBO, Candida) are not the same. Consequently, what works for one person (or even a majority of people) may not be the best for you. Before we take a look at some of the options, let's talk about some principles that I believe should always apply.

Some of the biggest offenders in the Standard American Diet (SAD) are processed foods, artificial sweeteners, artificial flavors, artificial food coloring/dyes, and sugar/sweets. Among these are foods that contain high fructose corn syrup (HFCS), partially hydrogenated oils, genetically modified organisms (GMOs), antibiotics, and pesticides. Also, some might be surprised to learn that excess fructose (eating too much fruit) can have the same negative effect on our liver as HFCS.

Next, let's chat about...yes, I'm going there, SUGAR! Sorry, guys and gals, but sugar is not good for our waistlines or our guts and immune systems. When we eat, we typically see a spike in insulin, but when our meal includes sugar, the added sugar sets us up for a cycle of negative effects. You may have heard the phrase, "Fat doesn't make you fat, sugar makes you fat." After everything that I have learned, I believe there is truth in that statement. However, we will talk more on insulin in a future chapter, but for now, let's carry on.

If you enjoy any of these foods on a daily basis, I'm sure you're ready to ditch this book, but hang in there with me. I believe knowledge is power, and if we want to truly be at our optimal, we need to take a look at how all of these foods are affecting us. Yes, processed foods are convenient, but for how long? Eventually, you will have to pay the price of what you're fueling your body with...whether that be in decreased energy or the havoc that all the processed foods are wreaking on your gut health and immune system, and in turn your thyroid and hormones. Foods that are highly processed cause faulty messaging to the brain, and our brains don't get the message that we are full. Plus, processed and artificial foods/flavors/colors are filled with chemicals which tend to disrupt our endocrine systems.

Additionally, in my research on what to eat when you have Candida, I found JJ Virgin's explanation of how we process sugar and carbs extremely helpful. As a whole, we have been taught to look at foods according to the glycemic index (GI) when making food choices. However, we need to take a closer look at both the amount of food (glycemic load) and how it's processed by the body. Essentially, the glycemic index measures how the foods we eat affect our blood sugar levels, but it's skewed based on how much we eat and the type of sugar (e.g., fructose...fruit). Fructose does not raise your blood sugar or insulin, but JJ Virgin stated that, "When you eat fructose, you bypass every one of your body's satiety safety nets, and your system functions in reverse. Your appetite switch is pegged in the on position, and it causes you to overeat. And worse yet, you're storing that fructose as fat." So, despite struggling with additional weight gain, it leaves us hungry, too. This is why it's important to know how food affects us when we are looking to reach our optimal state. I think it's more difficult to be spunky if we are struggling with our weight...or having cravings and feeling hungry. Plus, we have to be intentional, but it is possible to eat REAL, healthy foods that are tasty and delicious!

This is not a comprehensive list, but let's take a look at some of the healthier, popular eating plans:

- Whole 30
- Paleo
- Autoimmune Paleo (AIP)
- Mediterranean
- Low FODMAP
- Anti-Candida Diet (like a restricted Paleo)
- Adrenal Reset Diet
- Metabolism Reset Diet
- Body Ecology Diet
- Virgin Diet or Sugar Impact Diet
- Vegan
- Vegetarian
- Ketogenic (Keto)
- Intermittent Fasting

Some of the diets listed above may not be familiar to you, but I'm sure that you have at least heard of a few of them. I believe all of these diet protocols have health benefits and could be adopted as a daily eating plan. However, I want to quickly discuss why certain plans (or at least certain variations of some plans) might be beneficial for some but not everyone. Many of these are very similar in their principles, and I'm not going to take time to break them all down, but I would encourage you to always research the science behind a diet before initiating it. Plus, at various times we might need to adopt a temporary plan to achieve a specific goal (e.g., weight loss, eliminating food intolerances, controlling Candida) before returning to our normal plan.

I believe the Ketogenic plan (Keto) is a good example to explain how a plan (or variations of this plan) can be beneficial for many, but may not be for all. There are several variations of the Keto diet...and many adapt it to fit within their lifestyle, and some versions are healthy...and some are not so healthy. I will not be going into all of the specifics, so if you have never heard about the Keto diet or if you want to learn more about a healthier Keto diet, I would recommend checking out information from some of the top advocates and educators on this topic, like Thomas DeLaur; Dr. David Jockers DNM, DC, MS; Dr. Eric Berg, DC; and Dr. Josh Axe, DC, DNM, CNS. They share a lot of science behind its validity of use and even share its effect on the thyroid. Some experts argue that someone who is highly active or has thyroid problems needs to eat at least 50 grams of carbohydrates per day to support thyroid functioning; however, others suggest that the change in thyroid levels reflects improved thyroid sensitivity. So, it appears that some may do well due to positive effects of being in nutritional ketosis. In a nutshell, ketosis causes a decrease in T3 levels (the active thyroid hormone), so those who suffer from thyroid disease may need to adapt their diet accordingly if they are not seeing these beneficial effects with their weight and overall health. The thyroid is particularly sensitive to nutritional deficiencies so there is the potential that ketosis and low-carb diets can have a negative impact on our thyroids. However, with this in mind, remember what I said about the variations with the Keto diet. There are options to adapt a HEALTHY (key word) Keto diet to make it more thyroid friendly. Raising carbohydrate intake slightly is one option or carb cycling or boosting fat intake are additional options that may help make it more doable. Another suggestion is to look into options such as Dr. Anna Cabeca's Keto-Green™ diet and lifestyle. Dr. Cabeca is the author of a newly released book, *The Hormone Fix*, and in a recent blog post she explained the difference between a typical Keto diet and her Keto-Green program and why her program is beneficial for women with thyroid disease. After I give a brief overview of the key differences, you will see why I would direct you more to this style of Keto. The key differences...alkaline diet and lifestyle (less inflammation), removes food intolerances, avoids environmental toxins, and includes lifestyle changes that positively impact the thyroid (better sleep, stress management, adrenal support...and improving gut health). Do you see why I would steer you more towards this type of Keto?! The biggest key in choosing an eating plan is to pay attention to your body and choose a diet that works best for you! More importantly, make sure your diet is nutrient-dense and meets your specific needs. Eat to fuel and nourish your body.

•   •   •

FIND YOUR SPUNK TIP:
Consider Starting with an Elimination Diet & Listen to Your Body

•   •   •

I honestly believe, as mentioned in the previous chapter, that the biggest game changer is removing food intolerances from our diets. If you don't know what foods you may be sensitive to, you could opt for a food sensitivity test, as discussed previously, or begin with an elimination diet, like the Autoimmune Paleo Diet (AIP). The most common food intolerances are gluten, dairy, soy, grains (especially corn), nightshades (e.g., potatoes, tomatoes, and peppers), eggs, nuts, and seeds. Two goitrogenic foods that I would highly recommend avoiding are soy and canola oil. Both are typically made from genetically modified organism (GMO) crops, and soy is believed to play a role in blocking the activity of the TPO enzyme and is linked to autoimmune thyroiditis. There is a debate on cruciferous veggies (e.g., broccoli, cauliflower, cabbage), but it appears that unless you have a sensitivity to them they should be okay in small amounts...preferably cooked or fermented. Additionally, if you are without a thyroid, like myself, then the goitrogenic foods rule does not apply, but it's still good to avoid non-fermented soy and canola/vegetable oil. In addition, a good general rule for all is to decrease the intake of processed foods, sugar, and carbohydrates and just eat REAL food! Foods with less ingredients are healthier for us and easier to digest. Eating processed, chemically-laden foods are stressful on our systems. The foods we eat can literally play a part in hurting or healing our guts. Plus, don't be afraid to eat healthy fats like coconut, olive, avocado, and macadamia nut oils and healthy proteins.

I personally prefer to include a little bit of carb cycling and intermittent fasting. I suppose I have days where I'm mainly eating a healthy Keto diet, but it is not a diet I follow on a daily basis. However, when following the Anti-Candida and Low FODMAPS diet I was basically following the Keto diet. I'm not a diehard in any of these approaches because I believe the biggest key is to eat a diverse diet. I do, however, like to give myself a decent break between dinner and breakfast (and I do workout first thing in the morning on an empty stomach...or very minimal calories). I would say I'm typically in the 14- to 15-hour range between dinner and breakfast, but it definitely varies. However, I am not one to skip breakfast and wait until lunch. I prefer to have a nutrient dense shake for breakfast (with protein, fiber, and fat), and I always squeeze three meals in each day. I would much rather eat an early dinner, and let it have plenty of time to settle before I go to bed. This is definitely a personal preference though...you do YOU! Also, I'm not afraid of healthy fats, and I eat tons of veggies (typically flavored with healthy oils) and each meal includes protein, fiber, and fat...which I believe is the best combo for a healthy meal!

On a final note, before we move on, I did want to mention a tidbit of advice I learned from Dr. Alan Christianson regarding carbs. Dr. Christianson is the author of *The Adrenal Reset Diet* and *The Metabolism Reset Diet* books. He recommended including small portions (¼ - 1 cup, per meal) of good carbs (e.g., beets, parsnips, turnips, lentils, black beans, chickpeas, quinoa, buckwheat, and black rice) because they are more stable. Bad carbs, like sugary foods make your blood sugar unstable and create extra cortisol. The good carbs take longer to absorb and provide more steady energy and help stave off hunger longer. He does note that you should stay closer to the lower recommended amount of carbs during times when you are less active or trying to lose weight, but suggests not going lower than this amount.

Again, this comes back to listening to your body! It WILL tell you when it's not happy, whether that be an upset stomach, acne, hives, or even achy joints. Like I mentioned in the intro, my doctor said that food intolerances are messengers, but so are common symptoms that many of us ignore or excuse as just part of the aging process. So, first we eliminate the top food offenders, next we keep track of our foods by journaling, then we listen to our bodies (and after a time begin reintroducing foods). From there we determine a plan.

Chapter 6

Ditch the Gunk in Your Gut

Our gut is our second brain, and it's SO important to make sure we take care of it because it can have a huge impact on our overall health! A sluggish gut can mess with our hormones and throw our systems out-of-whack. A "leaky" gut can lead to even bigger issues! Sadly, there is likely a large number of us suffering from a leaky gut, but most are unaware of it. What is leaky gut? Basically, it's exactly what it sounds like, certain factors such as a poor diet, an unhealthy balance of the good and bad bugs in our gut, stress, hormone imbalances, and issues with unbalanced blood sugar levels can damage our intestinal wall lining, which then allows toxins, food particles, and bacteria to "leak" out into our bloodstream. No one is exempt, but it's an area that we have a lot of control over. Additionally, our gut is not only our "second brain." but it plays a big role in our immunity (approximately 80%), so if we are stuffing it with junk, how do we expect it to stay healthy and fight for us? Think of it this way, pretend your gut is an Olympic athlete getting ready for a competition (maybe even the Olympics). How do you think he/she would perform if he/she ate a lot of candy and junk food right before his/her competition? My guess is that he/she wouldn't have the appropriate fuel/energy to fight for victory. Same goes for our guts! If we want our guts to fight against sickness and disease (or whatever we are battling), wouldn't you want it to be in fighting shape?

I also like to think about food as being fuel for our bodies. If we put bad fuel in, how is it supposed to run properly? If you put bad gas in a car...or artificial gas, what is going to happen? It's either going to have difficulty running or not run at all. Do we expect foods that have been altered from their original state to nourish and fuel us as the real deal? I, for one, can attest to the difference in how I feel when I eat the junk versus nutrient-dense foods. If you have ever done a good detox, then you know how much energy you can gain by ridding the body of all the junk that has been clogging it up...and how much energy you can gain when you start fueling up on nutrient-dense foods. It's just like when you flush out bad gas from your tank and fill it with good gas, you're good to go!

Let me give you a personal example. For about a year and a half, I have dealt with a lot of bloating and weight gain despite trying to do all of the "right" things. However, it wasn't until I had blood work done that I was able to figure out what was going on. I discovered that my body was trying to fight Candida (a yeast infection, which for me was internal...so I couldn't see it). This issue with Candida is that it feeds on sugar and carbs, and if you don't have enough "good bugs" in your system, the Candida can take over. The hard thing is that you end up craving the very things you shouldn't eat! Plus, my labs revealed that my immunity was down because it was trying to fight the Candida, and I showed evidence of liver damage. However, once I figured out what was going on, I was able to feed my body what it needed (including getting more Omega-3 and probiotics) while avoiding those foods that were feeding the Candida to begin healing my gut and my liver. Everything was going well, and then I hit a stumbling block when introducing more foods back into my diet. All of a sudden, I started reacting with hives all over my stomach and the bloating was back! Not cool! Well, we will talk more about this in a bit, but first let's talk about what makes up our gut.

"All disease begins in the gut"
-Hippocrates, father of western medicine

Our gut is comprised of a whole series of microbes that are either working for us or against us. A couple of years ago, I was introduced to the term microbiome. Have you heard of it? Our gut microbiome is the trillions of bacteria (good and bad), fungi, or viruses that live within our digestive tract, and it's essentially in charge of our immune system and health. The greater the diversity of our microbiome, the better. We have and need both good and bad bugs; however, we need to make sure we have more "good bugs" than "bad bugs." The foods we eat have a huge impact on the diversity of our microbiome. Plus, a poor diet, stress, antibiotic usage and other factors can negatively affect our ratio of good versus bad bugs. When there is an imbalance in the bacteria in our gut, it leads to gut dysbiosis (aka our gut bacteria is out-of-whack). Those suffering from gut dysbiosis typically present with one or more of the following signs/symptoms:

- Bloating, gas, constipation, diarrhea
- Food allergies or intolerances
- Skin problems, such as eczema and acne
- Mood swings, anxiety, or depression
- Suppressed immune (or autoimmune issues)
- Fatigue
- Weight gain
- Cravings (typically sugar)
- Bad breath

If you begin to research information on our microbiome, you will discover that gut health has a connection to thyroid health. It is also linked to many other conditions, including autoimmune disease and even heart health. In fact, Dr. Carel Le Roux believes that our gut is responsible for hormonal control in the body, and we should start focusing on the gut when treating many hormonal imbalances and diseases, including type-1 and type-2 diabetes (Society of Endocrinology, 2019). We will dive deeper into hormonal balance in an upcoming chapter. I don't know about you, but I find it fascinating how our guts have so much control over our health. I wish I had learned all of this information a long time ago...which is now why I am sharing it with you.

Before we move on, let's talk about the liver's role in the whole process...which is actually pretty significant. Our liver is our body's key organ for detoxification. Every product that we use or consume, including chemicals in the air that we breathe, is filtered through our liver. It helps remove and clean toxins and heavy metals out of our blood. If our liver is healthy and working at its best capability, then our bodies will perform optimally at removing toxins. However, due to the large amount of toxins we face on a daily basis, we place a large demand on our livers. So, consider what happens when our liver gets bogged down with an excess of toxins. The liver is our biggest internal organ and it has many jobs, so if we bog down our liver or cause damage, then it will have a huge impact on our overall health.

Additionally, we've already discussed "leaky gut", but Dr. Christianson believes we can also have "leaky livers." He mentioned that this is where the liver is essentially dumping energy as it overflows, storing it as fat. Interestingly, Dr. Christianson referred to diabetes as a disease of the liver. He believes we can repair our liver, stop storing fat, and lose weight naturally with a proper liver detox. Consequently, there are huge gains that we can make regarding our health by focusing on keeping our liver healthy because a large part of our well-being depends on the state of our liver health.

• • •

FIND YOUR SPUNK TIP:
Eat Pre- & Probiotic Rich Foods

• • •

If you're like me, then you're probably wondering what you need to do to balance your gut bacteria. I say balance because although it would be nice to never have to deal with "bad" bugs, our bodies actually need a healthy balance of both. The best step we can take is to first figure out the root cause of the imbalance. In fact, many of the "ditch" items in this book can play a role towards an imbalanced microbiome. In addition, depending on the severity of your symptoms or imbalances, it may be necessary to seek out a holistic practitioner for additional help.

When you have an unhealthy gut, most typical protocols recommend starting with a cleanse/detox (which may also include coffee enemas or colonic hydrotherapy). However, when doing a cleanse, it is important to make sure to include the correct nutrients to ensure that all of the toxins are removed from our bodies. For instance, amino acids play a key role in clearing toxins, so we need to make sure to include clean protein when detoxing. When I was researching the best methods for detoxing our livers, I learned that we need to be careful about doing juice based cleanses (without protein) because while they are beneficial for freeing up the toxins in our bodies, they need protein to complete the job. We do want to free up the toxins, but even more importantly, we want to remove them from our systems. If we free them up and don't flush them out then they are free to attack...and we don't want that!!! That would leave us in worse shape than when we started. Additionally, when we think of detoxing, we often think of a once a year (or at most quarterly) activity. However, detoxing is a practice that we should incorporate every day. By including daily habits that help to detox our bodies, we can minimize the buildup of toxins in our guts/liver.

Next, once we have effectively cleansed our bodies, what types of foods should we eat? In all of my research, there seemed to be a consensus on the following types of foods: fermented foods/vegetables, garlic, onion, bone broth, and high-fiber foods. Interestingly enough, these foods are rich in sulfur...which we will discuss in a bit. While many may turn their noses up to the thought of eating fermented veggies, it is possible to adjust to the taste within a few days. So, don't get discouraged if the thought of fermented foods doesn't appeal to you...there is hope! I finally gave them a try and I'm hooked! I started with a brand I found in the refrigerated section at Whole Foods. I saw that there was a jar of fermented vegetables seasoned with curry, so I figured that would be a good place to start. The vegetables can be added to a salad or you can add a little healthy oil to change the taste a bit, so you can play with the flavor a little. Fermented pickles might be another good place to start. What do you think? Are you willing to give it a try?

Some of the best ways we can take care of our gut is to eliminate food intolerances, make healthier changes to our diets, lower our stress levels, get plenty of sleep, avoid toxins (endocrine disruptors), stay hydrated, and take pre- and probiotics. It all essentially comes down to the health of our guts. So, while eating healthy, nutrient dense foods are an important piece, we also want to make sure we have a healthy gut microbiome. When we have more bad bacteria than good bacteria we start to have issues. So, the gut is a good place to start when we are seeking optimal health...and we need to work to replace the bad bacteria with the good. We want to make sure the good outnumbers the bad!

While all the points we have discussed will help us improve our gut health, we also need to make sure we are giving ourselves an extra boost. In my research, I found some key foods and supplements that proved to be helpful in restoring my gut microbiome. So, along with following the guidelines above (with ditching the bad and adding the good), here are the best additions I have made to my diet (along with some key info I learned about them):

- A good probiotic!
- Coconut Kefir or Kefir Water
- Fermented Vegetables
- Prebiotic Fibers
- Apple Cider Vinegar
- Digestive Enzymes
- Phytonutrient dense foods - Polyphenols
- Omega-3s
- Coconut oil/MCTs
- Bone Broth

- Sulfur-rich foods/supplements
- Supplements and vitality essential oils for gut and liver support

I wish I had started taking probiotics earlier so that my body would have had a better chance of stopping the Candida before it started, but I am now taking it faithfully every day and working to build up the good bacteria in my gut. Also, did you know that if you've had your appendix removed that it's even more important for you to make sure to feed your body with probiotics? They used to think that there wasn't a purpose for the appendix, but they have since discovered that it's like a holding tank for extra good bacteria. So, if you are like me and you are missing your appendix, make sure to load up on good probiotics!!! We have to be extra diligent in making sure we are replenishing the good bacteria in our gut since we don't have a reserve available. Though, probiotics are beneficial for everyone.

Coconut kefir, kefir water, and fermented vegetables are also a good way to get good bacteria into our guts. Since fermented veggies help to eat up the bad stuff that we eat, we can include them with a couple of our meals each day. I haven't been able to get my family to try fermented veggies, but they do enjoy the coconut water kefir (we like the Kevita brand). Another fermented beverage that many drink, Kombucha, is not recommended because of the wild yeast from the air, plus most varieties include higher amounts of sugar. Next, although apple cider vinegar (ACV) is fermented, it is thought to be more of a prebiotic. There are many benefits of consuming ACV, and I encourage you to do a little research to learn all about additional benefits. Aside from acting as a prebiotic fiber, it can also provide the stomach with additional acid to help breakdown the foods we eat. Believe it or not, it is more likely for people to have issues with low stomach acid as opposed to too much stomach acid. So, if you experience digestive issues you may actually need more acid instead of less. I typically use between one to three tablespoons a day. It can be taken as one serving in a glass of water or broken down into 3 teaspoon/tablespoon servings before/after each meal.

Prebiotics or prebiotic fibers are an awesome way to feed the good bacteria in the gut. I mentioned ACV above, which has apple pectin, but there are many types of prebiotic fibers. While the fiber may be indigestible to us they are actually quite beneficial for the "good bugs" in our gut. Have I grossed you out yet? I'm sure you love thinking about all the bugs in your gut feasting on the fibers you eat? Sorry, but you will have to trust me...this is a good thing! Wouldn't you rather feed the good than the bad? I like to think of it as fiber feeds the good, and sugar feeds the bad. Who's winning the war in your gut?

Before I move on, I want to give you a little lesson on prebiotic fibers. There are actually three different types, with the third being somewhat interesting, and one that I've recently been learning more about. The three types are as follows:

- Insoluble fiber (e.g., bran)
- Soluble fiber (e.g., inulin, pectins, oats, psyllium husk)
- Resistant Starch (RS) (e.g., green banana flour and potato starch)

The different types of fiber feed on different species of gut bacteria, but I want to talk a little bit more about resistant starch. Resistant starch wasn't really on my radar before researching how to heal my gut, but I have to say that it's amazing what you can learn when you start researching! It's honestly quite fascinating how our body interacts with different types of food...the items we digest and those we don't. I became more aware of resistant starches when Dr. Alan Christianson made the announcement about his new book, *The Metabolism Reset Diet* (which has since been released and I've already bought and read it). Although I have not yet done his 28-day reset diet, I have learned some interesting information about taking care of our liver. The liver is truly the key to a healthy metabolism.

So, what is resistant starch and why should we add this carbohydrate to our diets? Yes, it is a carbohydrate, but hang on while I explain how it is metabolized differently in our bodies. While most carbohydrates are broken down and absorbed as glucose by the time they reach the small intestines, resistant starches (and starch digestion products) pass right through the small intestines without being digested and absorbed and go straight to the large intestines (aka colon). Once it arrives in the colon, it acts as a prebiotic and helps to feed the good bugs in our gut (and turns the RS into short chain fatty acids). In turn, RS is beneficial for both gut health and liver functioning. Plus, it can have additional positive effects, such as improved blood sugar regulation and a decrease in both adiposity and visceral fat.

There are actually four different kinds of resistant starches, but I'm not going to get into the nitty gritty of the different types since most people just want a list of foods that include them. However, aside from the man-made version, you will find RS in grains, seeds and legumes (bound within fibrous cell walls and does not get broken down in the small intestines), some starchy foods (e.g., raw potatoes and green bananas), and certain digestible carbs that can turn into RS if cooked then cooled (e.g., rice and potatoes). Plus, the different types can coexist in the same food, and the amount of resistant starch is dependent on factors like ripeness or how the foods are prepared. RS is typically highest in raw form. For instance, I mentioned green bananas above, which would mean an unripe banana because once it ripens and turns yellow it loses the resistant starch and becomes a regular starch. If you would like to look at a more comprehensive list of resistant starch sources, a link can be found in the appendix.

Why would we want to add it to our diets? I haven't done enough research to determine if resistant starch has been shown to have a significant effect on weight loss, but from what I have seen it does not appear to increase weight. Studies have shown that it helps to lower whole body and visceral fat...you know the fat that surrounds our organs (and even happens with thin people). In fact, according to Dr. Higgins' report in the *Critical Reviews in Food Science and Nutrition* journal, "The magnitude of these changes in adiposity are very large and sufficient to independently improve insulin sensitivity, and reduce the risk of diabetes, CVD [Cardiovascular Disease], and certain cancers." So, before you consider ditching all carbs, you may want to consider keeping resistant starch in your arsenal.

Next, our bodies make some digestive enzymes, but not typically enough to truly digest what we eat, and the amount of enzymes we produce decreases as we age. Therefore, it's good to include digestive enzymes in our daily routine. Digestive enzymes take the burden off of our digestive tract and help breakdown the proteins, fats, and carbohydrates. There are different enzymes to breakdown the separate macronutrients, so we want to make sure we are taking enzymes that are breaking down the fats and protein that we are eating. Although, we don't want to break down our carbs too quickly. If we're eating a healthy diet, we don't need to worry about the carbohydrate enzyme as much. There are many different types of enzymes, but the following are the top enzymes for each macronutrient group:

- Protein - Protease
- Fat - Lipase
- Carbs - Amylase

I should also note that if you have had your gallbladder removed, I've heard that digestive enzymes are a must! Similar to how those of us without an appendix need to make sure to supplement with probiotics, individuals without a gallbladder require added digestive enzymes (and it sounds like ox bile, too) to help break down fat.

Next, I think many know the importance of eating a diet rich in phytonutrient dense foods. "Phyto" refers to the Greek word for plant, so we are essentially talking about a diet high in fruits and vegetables. More specifically, we want foods that are high in polyphenols. Polyphenols are the naturally-occurring compounds that are found in plant foods such as fruits and vegetables, herbs (e.g., oregano), spices (e.g., cloves), along with dark chocolate, coffee/tea, and wine. If you would like to check out what types of foods are rich in polyphenols, a link that includes the top 100 richest foods in polyphenols can be found in the appendix. Polyphenols are great for our gut microbiome. Consuming polyphenols is a great way to increase good bacteria in our guts along with decreasing the bad bacteria. It is beneficial for balancing our gut bacteria. Therefore, we want to make sure our diet is rich in polyphenols and plant-based foods.

Additionally, Omega-3s have been noted to have a beneficial effect on our gut microbiome as well. According to a study published in the *International Journal of Molecular Science*, when enough Omega-3s were consumed, they have been shown to produce greater microbial diversity along with increasing the production of short-chain fatty acids (anti-inflammatory compounds). Also, animal studies revealed that Omega-3s appear to help maintain the integrity of the intestinal wall as well as interact with host immune cells.

I should mention that up until now we've been discussing the good and bad bacteria in the gut, but as I previously mentioned, one of the biggest issues facing many of us today is leaky gut. Despite being a fairly healthy eater, I believe my gut had become "leaky" years ago, and I just didn't know it. It's hard to "fix" something when you don't know that it's "broken." So, this is most likely the cause of the food intolerances I began to experience over the years...which progressed fairly significantly within the last year. This basically opened the door for issues such as the Candida overgrowth and hives after eating certain foods. Consequently, it's important to note that even people who adopt a healthier eating pattern still have the potential for developing gut issues. Therefore, it's important to know steps to take to help prevent leaky gut, but it's also important to know the typical signs and symptoms along with steps you can take to heal a leaky gut. Trust me, your gut and body will thank you!

Interestingly, many of the foods already mentioned, along with two that we have yet to discuss (coconut/MCT oil and bone broth), are also recommended for those dealing with leaky gut. So, by taking steps to improve our microbiome we may also improve a leaky gut. However, when choosing foods or supplements, the key is to remember that we all react differently to various foods. So, just like with our diets, we need to pay attention to our own bodies and see how we respond to the different foods. For instance, my dad has an allergy to bananas, so he is not going to use green banana flour as a resistant starch as a prebiotic fiber to boost good bugs in his system. This would actually have a negative impact on his gut health.

Okay, now onto coconut oil and bone broth! Both coconut (and MCT) oil and bone broth are beneficial for our gut health. Coconut oil is rich in lauric acid, which is known to have powerful anti-microbial agents that help to kill off yeast and bad bacteria in the gut. Plus, the medium chain triglycerides (MCTs) play a role in helping to heal the gut lining. Bone broth has nutrients such as bone marrow that helps to support our cells and immune system. It is one of the first foods that was recommended to me after I learned I was dealing with Candida and SIBO...and a coinciding leaky gut. So, both coconut oil and bone broth have been a big part of my diet for the past several months due to their amazing benefits.

When it comes to fighting candida the natural way, several holistic doctors recommend including caprylic acid (one of the fatty acids found in coconut oil). Candida is a condition that occurs when an overgrowth of yeast fungus develops in your gut. Therefore, because caprylic acid acts as a natural yeast-fighting agent, it is believed that it can penetrate the cell membranes of Candida yeast cells and cause them to die off, detoxifying the digestive tract and speeding up the healing process. If you want more bang for your buck, you can take caprylic acid and Omega-3 (fish oil supplements) in combination. This powerhouse duo is thought to be one of the best supplemental supports for conditions such as Candida.

Additionally, since we mentioned that the liver was the main detox organ, we can't forget to focus some attention on this beloved organ. Did you know that it's the largest of our internal organs? I honestly never thought about it before, but now with everything that I'm learning, everything seems to lead back to the liver. When you think about all that the liver has to do, this makes sense. The scary part is that many people probably have some damage to their liver, and they just don't know it. This was the case for me. I freaked out when my blood test revealed I had some damage to my liver. However, I was relieved when I learned that we can regenerate our livers...provided we don't wait too long. This put me on a mission to discover how to heal my liver! If you haven't figured out yet...I'm a fighter, very tenacious, and I don't give up!!!

So, what can we do to support our liver? Some of the tips that I learned didn't apply to me, but I will share them in case they help you. For instance, one that I'm sure most of you are aware of is that alcohol and medications such as acetaminophen are hard on the liver (and the combo is worse). Plus, the toxic chemicals and endocrine disruptors (including the use of plastic products) can place a large demand on the liver. However, a new one for me was fructose, and I'm not just talking about High Fructose Corn Syrup, this includes yummy, delicious, pure fruit. Yes, fruit is a healthy food, but when we consume a large amount of it, it can also place an extra burden on our livers. I personally have been trying to limit my fruit intake to one or two servings a day. Fortunately, this correlates with the items we have already talked about ditching. Next, as far as what we can do to help support our liver, the biggest key is to increase glutathione, which is the main antioxidant for the liver. Glutathione plays a role in preventing cellular damage and detoxing. They say it doesn't really benefit us to take a glutathione supplement, but we can eat foods that help to increase glutathione. The best foods are those that are rich in sulfur, which include garlic and onions, cruciferous veggies and dark leafy greens, whey protein, eggs, and protein-rich foods. Organic and grass-fed foods/meats are best.

Lastly, in general I believe it's a good idea to continually clean out the toxins that accumulate in our bodies to protect both our liver and our gut. We can do things daily to detox, but I would also encourage you to consider looking into doing routine cleanses (for colon, kidneys, and liver). Even if you are trying to avoid toxins in your food choices and personal care products, we are still exposed to them through our environment, and we can't always avoid them in the foods that we consume. So, periodic cleanses will help flush out our systems and reset our bodies. However, one important lesson that I've learned this past year is that protein is necessary for the cleansing process. So, I would keep this in mind when choosing a specific cleanse to follow. Ditching the gunk in our gut is vital to our health!!!

Chapter 7

Ditch Imbalances

I have to tell you that I thought about calling this chapter, *Ditch the Resistance* because I was thinking about weight-loss resistance, insulin resistance, leptin resistance, and even thyroid resistance. I thought about doing a cute *Star Wars* analogy…as we fight to battle our own "resistance(s)." However, finding balance includes more than just these resistances, so I decided to stick with ditching imbalances to fully encompass the imbalances we face on a daily basis. The biggest imbalances we encounter are hormone imbalances (the resistances mentioned above…and more) and an out of balance schedule (aka circadian rhythm). Any kind of imbalance can throw us off kilter. Optimal and imbalance don't go together. So, let's talk a little bit about these imbalances.

First, erratic life and work schedules can create a huge imbalance with our Circadian rhythm, which can also affect our hormones and weight. An equation Dr. Suhas Kshirsagar (2018) mentioned in his online yoga training, *Yoga, Ayurveda & Lifestyle Medicine: The Amazing Healing Power of Daily Habits,* paints a very clear picture of how our habits affect us. He said, "Sleep late = Gain weight; Eat late = Gain weight." Plus, he mentioned that Sleep = Healing. Dr. Kshirsagar believes that if we change our schedule we can change our life. He mentioned that the blue light of our electronic gadgets within an hour before bed or upon waking can disrupt our Circadian rhythms due to the effect that blue light has on both melatonin and cortisol levels. Blue light affects melatonin release in the evenings and increases cortisol levels in the morning. Often, we follow a schedule that is not optimal for thriving at our best. I will share more about Dr. Kshiragar's tips in a bit.

Next, I think we all know what out-of-balance hormones does to our bodies. Unfortunately, it's not just one hormone we need to focus on, but several hormones that all play in symphony with each other. We need to make sure all of our hormones are in balance. If one is off (e.g., estrogen dominance), it can have a HUGE impact on thyroid levels, and our overall health. So, it's important to look at the big picture. I love the analogy Dr. Sara Gottfried used to explain how hormones work together (and I found it after I used the symphony analogy...which is probably why I liked her wording). She stated, "Your hormones exist in a delicate balance, playing alongside one another like instruments in an orchestra. Throughout the day your hormones fluctuate in rhythms, like crescendos of a symphony. Each hormone is like a specific instrument that must play on time and in rhythm with your other hormones. Together, your hormones create a beautiful harmony – your stable sense of wellbeing." She also added, "Whenever one of your hormones is out of tune, you feel it. Your rhythm and flow are affected. Eventually, a hormone out of rhythm affects those it interacts with and can set off a cascade of negative consequences. Because of the interconnectedness of your hormones, you can go from feeling totally fine one day to feeling completely off the next." Is that not a beautiful analogy?

As mentioned above, hormone imbalance is complex, so I want to break it down into some of the key factors and try to give a brief description/explanation of each one without going into a full-on anatomy lesson. If you are like me and like all the science and facts, consider doing a more in depth search, along with looking up some of the hormone experts listed in the appendix. I personally find all of the information fascinating, but I know many just want a simple breakdown...so I will do my best to keep it concise. The imbalances I want to touch on are: thyroid, insulin resistance, leptin resistance, and estrogen dominance. Plus, I will discuss the connection between all of these and provide additional information on cortisol, progesterone, estrogen, and thyroid hormone...and what is happening as we approach (or are dealing with) menopause.

First, I would like to do a quick break down of the endocrine system...what it is and a little about the hierarchy of the endocrine glands. I hope that I am able to provide you with enough information to allow you to get a good picture of how the system interplays with each other. The endocrine system is a complex system that consists of several different glands that each produce their own hormone(s). Some of these glands are well known, but others are less commonly known. The endocrine glands produce hormones that are released into our bloodstream and are carried to specific tissues or organs where they perform a given task (e.g., produce another hormone, cause a behavioral or other type of response, or change metabolism). The key glands of the endocrine system include the following: hypothalamus, pituitary, thyroid, adrenals, pancreas, and sex hormones. All of the glands affect each other, either directly or indirectly, which is why supporting our endocrine system and balancing hormones is very important. Additionally, since we just talked about our gut and liver health, I believe it's important to mention that our gut microbiome and liver play key roles in our endocrine system functioning. So, let's take a quick walk through of these key areas.

Let's start at the top and discuss the role of the hypothalamus. The hypothalamus is located deep in the center of the brain...in the middle of the limbic system, and it receives chemical signals through the nervous system (via blood and electrical signals) to keep it updated on the condition and needs of the body. It is considered the primary regulatory center of the body, and it helps regulate the metabolic functions of the body. The limbic system is the area of our brain that controls our basic emotions and drives (maternal/paternal instincts, hunger, sex, dominance). Did you know that our sense of smell is the only sense that has a direct connection to the limbic system? This means that the scents we inhale go directly to the brain (with no additional synapses). I'm sure you have had instances where you had a familiar scent from your past, and the scent brought back immediate memories of a certain time or place. I've heard that scents can show up instantly in the hypothalamus after they are held below the nose. So, the hypothalamus has a key role in our endocrine functioning, and scents can be influential too.

Next up is the pituitary gland. We briefly touched on this gland in chapter two, but now we will look at its overall responsibility. The pituitary gland is located at the base of the brain (connected to hypothalamus) and is about the size of a large pea. It receives messages from the hypothalamus and helps regulate the functions of other endocrine glands (thyroid, adrenals, and sex organs) by releasing hormones that carry messages from one cell to the other through your bloodstream. The pituitary gland is considered the "master gland" because it controls different processes, and it sends messages to other endocrine glands to stimulate or inhibit their own hormone production. There is a huge list of difficulties that can arise if we encounter any sort of injury or damage to the pituitary gland. So, although it is very small in size, it plays a major role in the endocrine process.

This brings us to the thyroid hormone, which is where my journey began many years ago when I was diagnosed with thyroid cancer. I had no clue of the significance our thyroid gland had back then, but you better believe I have done tons of research since then...along with living through the ups and downs of thyroid hormone regulation. Why am I so passionate about thyroid health and helping others find optimal thyroid levels? The reason is simple. I have lived through some very difficult experiences...with nerves going haywire throughout my entire body and almost unbearable pain at times that I hoped and prayed would go away. Well, I researched...found answers, and found practitioners willing to help me (and switched from my endocrinologist who refused to do full thyroid lab panels)...and my life CHANGED! Friends, if you are suffering, don't lose hope or give up! I believe your life can change too...and it is totally worth it! My deep desire now is to help others find their optimal wellness. If I can help others avoid the struggles I endured, even better! Plus, I want others to experience what it's like to find your "happy place" (aka optimal). I truly believe many people don't realize they have a thyroid hormone imbalance because they have been told their labs are within the "normal" range. To this I would question whether you have had a full thyroid panel and if you have a practitioner who is willing to listen and treat more to your symptoms rather than a lab test.

Our thyroid gland is responsible for boosting the metabolism of virtually every cell in our bodies. So, it has a huge effect on our metabolism, which plays a role in clearing toxins, our ability to fight disease or illness, it has a large impact on our reproductive health. For example, women who deal with thyroid disease often have issues with infertility and a progesterone deficiency. Consequently, by optimizing thyroid levels and functioning, we may help balance the entire endocrine system. However, when looking to optimize thyroid levels, we need to consider what is causing our levels to be unbalanced, and look for the underlying cause (not just changing dosing of medication). Plus, thyroid issues and symptoms vary from person-to-person so it is not a cookie-cutter disease. Many suffer from hypothyroidism (under active thyroid); however, others deal with the opposite, hyperthyroidism (overactive thyroid). In addition, these may be accompanied with an autoimmune disorder (e.g., Hashimoto's or Grave's Disease). Plus, those suffering from Hashimoto's disease may experience times of both hyper- and hypothyroidism due to the increase of thyroid hormone when the thyroid is being attacked. Unfortunately, this is then followed by a slow-down. There are common symptoms that most deal with, but some can be specific to the individual depending on cofactors that may be involved. However, the point of my book is not to teach you all about the different types of thyroid disease, but to teach you how to face it and thrive in spite of it. For those who might be wondering if this is something that they might be dealing with, I have included a couple of reference links in the appendix section with information on common symptoms. Plus, I have included links where you can find information on optimal thyroid lab values along with a list of my favorite people/sites that I like to follow, which include several thyroid/hormone experts.

Moving on to the adrenals gland, which has a close relationship with the thyroid. It produces several hormones, including a couple that you may have heard of...epinephrine (aka "adrenalin") and cortisol. Due to the number of hormones that are secreted by the adrenal glands, it is important to make sure it is well balanced and supported. The adrenal glands have an impact on our blood pressure, our reproductive system, hydration of the body via sodium/water retention, and several other processes. Plus, one very important lesson I have learned is that healthy adrenals is the key to easing gracefully into menopause. Yep, these glands are a pretty big deal!!!

Under times of stress, the adrenal glands release cortisol, the "stress hormone." Cortisol is a necessary hormone, and it is needed to help break down proteins in order for the liver to turn it into glucose during times of real emergencies. The issue arises when our bodies are in a constant state of stress, and the adrenal glands keep pumping out cortisol. This eventually leads to adrenal insufficiency or what some refer to as adrenal fatigue. When we are constantly bombarded with multiple types of stressors, including the toxic scents we breathe, our adrenal glands are constantly pumping out cortisol. This high stress (from both external and internal stressors) can cause a number of negative issues, including an increase in blood sugar levels, digestion problems, suppressed immune system, and weight gain. I had previously believed that our adrenals got tired and would "burn out," but I have since learned that it's a failure in communication (brain to adrenals). Due to the over-firing of the cortisol by the adrenals, the brain eventually stops sending messages to the adrenal glands, which is when many start experiencing symptoms such as fatigue. It kind of makes me think of the boy who cried wolf.

The best visual to help explain what happens to our adrenal glands when we have constant cortisol spikes is to use a smartphone as an analogy. If we are just using the phone normally then the battery seems to last a decent amount of time. However, consider what happens when you leave a bunch of apps open and play games or watch videos...what happens? If your smartphone is like mine, then the percentage of battery life drops considerably. We need the charging cord and either an outlet or battery charger to restore it to an optimal state. Well, our adrenals under constant stress are like a smartphone without a charger. Nothing is wrong with the phone, we just need to recharge it. Same goes with our adrenals...they don't "burn out" per se, they are just not receiving the message from the brain to keep firing. So, they essentially need a recharge. Therefore, we need to be mindful of daily stressors and lifestyle choices that place too much demand on our adrenal glands and cortisol production and remember to do daily activities to help recharge us.

Next in line is the pancreas...which actually belongs to two different systems, the endocrine and digestive. It secretes several hormones; however, the majority (more than 90%) of its cells work on the digestive side. Despite the small percentage of endocrine cells, it has a very important hormone that it secretes...insulin. Insulin is a hormone used to lower blood sugar and store body fat. It is made by the pancreas and is required for normal regulation of blood sugar levels (the amount of sugar glucose in the blood). Our cells use the glucose for energy, so if we don't have enough insulin (or are insulin resistance), the pancreas keeps trying to make more until it can no longer produce enough. If it reaches this point, our blood sugar rises. However, if our bodies are functioning optimally, insulin allows our cells to remove and use glucose from the blood as energy. Guess what happens to unused glucose? Unused glucose in the blood is eventually stored as body fat. An imbalance with insulin levels can wreak havoc on our bodies, so this is a key hormone to look at when seeking balance.

Did you know that every time we eat we cause our insulin to spike? It doesn't matter if we're eating a healthy snack or something on the opposite end of the spectrum, insulin levels will rise. If you research the effects of insulin, you will notice that an increase in insulin equals weight gain, and a decrease in insulin equals weight loss. So, all the diets that are telling us to eat every two hours to keep our metabolism revving are essentially forcing us to continuously spike our insulin levels. In my Health Coach training I learned that certain foods create a thermal effect when we eat, but it's not significant enough to consider them as a weight loss tool. So, I've come to realize, through both research and personal experience, that cutting out extra snacks can have a positive effect on our weight. This is due to both the decrease in calories and in insulin production.

Then, before we discuss the sex hormones (estrogen, progesterone, and testosterone), I want to talk about leptin and ghrelin, more specifically, leptin resistance, since it is similar to insulin resistance...and often goes hand in hand. The main reason I wanted to bring this up is because this information could be a game changer for many. Have you ever lost a lot of weight, but it came right back? If so, leptin may be the culprit. Ghrelin and leptin are hormones that control our appetite and weight regulation. I've heard ghrelin referred to as "GO" (the "hunger hormone") and leptin as "STOP" ("stop appetite hormone"). So, these hormones control whether you have an increase or decrease in hunger. Ghrelin sends the hunger signals...so we want to take steps to decrease this hormone if we want to lose weight...or increase it if we need to gain weight. Balance is the key! Remember our hormones work in symphony together and one imbalance can be like a tap of the first Domino, setting off a chain reaction.

So, what is leptin...and how do we become leptin resistant? Leptin, which is secreted from fat tissues, sends messages to the hypothalamus to signal when we are full (and tells us to STOP eating). However, since leptin is secreted by fat tissue it creates a cycle that can be hard to break. When you have higher amounts of body fat, you have more leptin; if there is too much then a similar situation to what happens with insulin resistance occurs with leptin. Basically, when too much is being secreted the message signals get all mixed up and our bodies no longer recognize that we are full...and so begins the cycle (we require more to feel full or satiated). We eat more, increase fat cells...which secretes more leptin. The easiest way for me to describe what happens with both insulin and leptin resistance is like what happens when you overload circuits, the circuits become overwhelmed. Everything is working fine when the system isn't overloaded, but once too much power is sent through the system, everything just shuts down. So, essentially, with leptin resistance, when our body's "circuit" has become overloaded with too much leptin being produced by the increase in fat cells, it stops sending messages to tell our brains that we are full. As you can see, leptin is a key component in our search for optimal balance.

Last, but not least, we have our sex organs, which secrete our sex hormones, which are typically the hormones that most people think about when talking about balancing hormones. Men and women have all three, we just have different proportions of each one. Again, the key is balance! There are several factors that can affect our sex hormone balance, including normal life changes like puberty, pregnancy, and menopause. For instance, Mary Shomon when addressing the issue of accompanying symptoms during the menopausal years stated that "it's not the lack of hormones that causes symptoms in most women. It's actually the up-and-down fluctuations in hormones, as well as imbalances in the ratio of hormones, that take place in the months and years before that last period that cause the most troublesome symptoms." So, it seems clear that it all comes back to balance.

As we age our sex hormone levels naturally decline. For women, the decline in estrogen and progesterone starts around our late thirties and Shomon indicated that it "is one of the most common triggers of a thyroid slow down." By the way, if you are a woman in your thirties (or older). I highly suggest picking up a copy of Mary Shomon's book, *The Thyroid Menopause Solution*. I will share a tiny glimpse from her book, but there is tons of valuable information to prepare us for menopause (or even to endure it better if you have already arrived). For instance, as I noted earlier, did you know that if you have thyroid issues it can send you into perimenopause far too early? Additionally, thyroid problems can make perimenopausal or menopausal symptoms worse...NOT cool!

In her book, Shomon dives into the reasons why older women or women who are menopausal have a higher chance for thyroid problems, which include, chronic stress, estrogen dominance, supplemental estrogen, and decreased progesterone. Sadly enough, Shomon stated that women who do not know they have thyroid problems, or are not receiving proper treatment, will most likely suffer more than other women. This honestly gives me a picture of a teeter totter…when you are teetering with someone around your same size, everything works smoothly, but once you switch out to someone who is heavier or smaller, the smoothness disappears and the struggles begin. The same goes for our hormones…too much stress, adrenals overwork…not enough progesterone, thyroid hormone decreases…too much estrogen, even more imbalance. We need to find the perfect symphony of balance.

Are you struggling to find balance? Did you know that estrogen dominance is one of the biggest issues we face with sex hormone imbalance? With all of the xenoestrogens that we face on a daily basis it makes it impossible to totally escape. As mentioned in the *Ditch the Endocrine Disruptors* chapter, these xenoestrogens are everywhere…in our food, personal care products, clothes, and furniture. Consider the symptoms of estrogen dominance, have you experienced any of these symptoms? Weight gain (primarily in the hips, waist, and thighs)…PMS or menstrual issues, such as abnormal bleeding…fibrocystic breasts, uterine fibroids, fatigue, loss of sex drive, or depression or anxiety? If so, Dr. Amy Myers indicated that these are the symptoms of estrogen dominance typically seen in women. For men, the symptoms typically involve enlarged breasts, sexual dysfunction, and infertility. Additionally, as if these symptoms aren't bad enough, estrogen dominance comes with some health risks, such as hormonal cancers, autoimmune disease, thyroid dysfunction, and Candida overgrowth. She explained that hormonal cancers (breast [men and women], uterine, ovarian, and prostate [men] are "associated with stored fat, which produces the most potent form of estrogen, estradiol." Dr. Myers explained that this type of estrogen is harmful and difficult for our bodies to detoxify, which leads to more circulating estrogen, which in turn affects thyroid hormone storage and conversion to the active form. Ummm...yikes!

For more detailed information, I recommend going to Amy Myers, MD's website (link in resources) to review a list of the typical causes of estrogen dominance...which happen to be many of the factors that we have already discussed (e.g., endocrine disruptors, gut dysbiosis, stress). In another post, Dr. Myers explains the science behind the estrogen dominance/gut dysbiosis connection. She stated that our "gut microbiome regulates circulating estrogen using an enzyme known as beta-glucuronidase." When we are out-of-balance in cases such as small intestinal bacterial overgrowth (SIBO), then we can't properly metabolize these estrogens via these enzymes...which can lead to estrogen dominance and other bigger issues.

Are you seeing how all of the various hormones interact with each other like a symphony, or how they can topple like a row of Dominos? Do you see why balance is crucial? How one imbalance can cause a myriad of issues? Now that we have an idea of what is going on, what can we do to support our hormones to achieve balance? Let's break it down below.

• • •

FIND YOUR SPUNK TIP:
Align Your Activities to the Dark and Sunlight...and Get Plenty of Sleep

• • •

One of the key steps we can take is to change our schedules to reset our Circadian rhythm. Dr. Kshirsagar's tips for resetting our Circadian rhythm are as follows:

- Don't touch electronic gadgets (blue light entertainment) at least an hour before bed and for one hour upon waking.
- Eat with the sunlight.
- Do a vigorous/brisk workout first thing before breakfast.
- Eliminate unwanted snacking.
- Align your activities to dark and sunlight.

He stresses that if we eat late or sleep late, we will most likely gain weight. Sounds like a chant, doesn't it? "Eat late, sleep late, gain weight!" Getting enough sleep and being mindful of when we eat can have a dramatic effect on helping to balance our hormones, too. Plus, his advice is good general practice and initiating these daily changes can have a beneficial impact on our health.

Additionally, many of the tips in this book are meant to provide helpful information on how to support our thyroid for optimal balance, so I won't repeat it all here. However, some key steps to finding optimal balance is to be your own advocate, have a full-thyroid panel performed, find a practitioner willing to help you find your optimal levels, avoid endocrine disruptors, take care of your gut/liver, and eat foods that support thyroid function (and avoid goitrogenic foods or food intolerances). Plus, aside from keeping our gut flora in a good place, we need to strive to find balance with all of our other hormones, so that it doesn't decrease thyroid functioning.

Additionally, if you are a fan/believer in the power of essential oils, did you know they can support your thyroid and endocrine system? Even though I don't have a thyroid, I use essential oils to support my endocrine system daily. As stated previously, scents can show up instantly in the hypothalamus after scents are held below the nose. So, don't be afraid to give pure essential oils a try, as they can play a big role in supporting our endocrine systems.

With our adrenal glands, it's vital that we take care of and nourish them. Since the hormones released by the adrenal glands are made from cholesterol, it makes sense that we would need to include fatty acids such as Omega-3s in our diets. I think when we start restricting these healthy fats from our bodies, it puts more stress on us and our adrenals. Additionally, B vitamins along with vitamin C and D seem to be the key vitamins to support your adrenals, so whenever possible choose foods that are rich in these vitamins and consider supplementing, if needed. I would highly recommend working with a holistic practitioner and checking lab levels before adding any new supplements to your regimen. Other supplements that I include in my diet that are beneficial for adrenal health, are probiotics (along with fermented veggies and coconut water kefir), ashwagandha (an adaptogen), and zinc. Plus, my practitioner recommended that I up my sea salt intake (I use Celtic sea salt). Oh, and another food that I know is good for the adrenal glands is sea veggies...which I still want to figure out how to include in my diet. I get them occasionally in one of the fermented vegetable brands that I buy, but I'm sure it's not enough to make a difference. Baby steps! Little by little I keep adding new foods to my diet. My practitioner has not recommended magnesium, but I have seen that recommended several times for those who may be experiencing fatigue from their adrenals. Other foods that are frequently recommended are greens and sulfur-rich vegetables (I love my greens and veggies!!!), coconut oil (add to morning shakes and use with veggies), avocados (I eat ½ to 1 avocado every day), grass-fed meats, and organ meats (haven't ventured into this one yet). Lastly, it's best to ditch the foods that make the adrenal glands work harder...added sugars (of any kind), white flour products, and gluten-containing grains.

Next, aside from nourishing our adrenals with the appropriate nutrients, one of the next best things we can do is to reduce stress. Stress is such a big issue that many of us deal with on a daily basis, and I believe it is one of the main contributors to the imbalances we face. For instance, let me give you an idea of how one hormone imbalance can cause a domino effect due to stress by looking at what can happen when we have high cortisol levels. If cortisol levels are high, it can deplete progesterone, which then in turn can affect thyroid levels and potentially even cause estrogen dominance. Say what?! I don't know about you, but that is just stressful thinking about it. Consequently, because we live in such a rushed society, we are constantly on the go, rushing from one activity to the other, and we often find it hard to hit the pause button and take time out for ourselves. So, with that being said, I'm going to make us hit the pause button right now because I believe this topic deserves more attention. We will come back to this topic soon...in the *Ditch the Stress* chapter, but for now, relax your shoulders and take a few deep breath and let your adrenal glands know they can take a break. Don't worry, we will talk more on this soon!

Next, how do we maintain and support healthy insulin levels? I believe the biggest key is to eat real food and give your body a break between meals to digest and break down the foods that we have eaten. Constantly spiking our blood sugar and insulin is stressful on our systems, so taking a break and cutting out extra snacking allows our bodies time to rest and heal. Intermittent fasting and a healthy Keto diet may help improve insulin levels as well. Additionally, by choosing to eat foods with a low-glycemic index rating, which take longer to break down and absorb, there is less chance for insulin spikes. Lastly, in addition to a healthy diet, exercise can have a beneficial effect on insulin resistance.

Leptin resistance, which often coexists with insulin resistance can be a stubborn one, but the good news is that it is possible to stop this vicious cycle of weight loss resistance by resetting leptin. From what I have read, it appears that in order to reset leptin resistance, one must follow the same protocol as you would with insulin resistance. It seems like most of the issues with weight gain involve too frequent spiking of certain hormones...cortisol, insulin, and leptin. So, we need to focus on reducing these spikes. The culprit? Foods that are high in sugar or high fructose sugar, or foods that quickly convert to sugar (carbs) are the biggest problem because they cause a more immediate spike...and the more frequently we eat during the day, the more spikes we will experience. So, when we cut down on these foods (or ditch them altogether), along with spacing out meals, so that our digestive system has time to recover...we avoid additional spikes. Intermittent fasting may also prove to be beneficial. I have personally found that by making sure that I am getting enough healthy fats, fiber, and protein at each meal, I am able to extend the time between each meal, and I have no difficulty fasting for around 15 hours between dinner and breakfast the next morning. Previously, I was on a schedule where I needed to eat every two hours...or I felt "hangry!" Ever have that feeling??? Plus, I would crave things like corn chips...and things that were not so healthy. However, once I started making changes...cutting out the foods with sugar (or that convert to sugar) and making sure I had my protein, fiber, and fat at each meal, my cravings...and the "hangry" feeling went away. I love that I don't have to worry about always having a snack on hand...and that I don't think about food all of the time!!! The good news is that this is not specific to me. I have read stories of how others have experienced the same. In a nutshell, when we stop allowing our leptin to spike (same goes with insulin) then we allow our body to reset, and then the brain will start to receive messages again helping us know that we are full...and to stop eating.

Have you ever noticed that you eat more when you are tired? Getting an adequate amount of sleep plays an important role in regulating both ghrelin and leptin. Reduced sleep has been shown to be a factor in weight gain, which might be due to the changes in our leptin and ghrelin levels when we don't get enough sleep. It typically causes a decrease in leptin and an increase in ghrelin (our hunger hormone). This is why you might find yourself snacking more on the days following a poor night's sleep. Sleep plays a huge part in our overall health and wellbeing...and it could be part of the key to helping you control your eating habits. So, let's move on to ghrelin!

How do we put the STOP on ghrelin (which is kind of like a gremlin)? In short, I believe there are four key areas that we need to focus on: diet, exercise, sleep, and stress. The issue with our diet lies more with dieting, especially when there is a severe calorie restriction. This is because it causes an increase in ghrelin output; however, processed foods can also interfere with the messaging pathway. Decreased sleep (as we already discussed) and stress also cause an increase of ghrelin. So, it makes sense that we would want to apply strategies to focus in on these key areas. I'm always preaching that you don't have to eat less, you just have to choose better options. Consequently, I believe the biggest effect can be made by including clean protein (vegan or grass-fed/organic meats), fiber, and healthy fats for all of our meals. We will talk more about sleep and reducing stress in the upcoming chapters, but both of these are vital if we want to find balance with leptin and ghrelin...and all of our other hormones. Lastly, it's not always my favorite, although short and quick, High Intensity Interval Training (HIIT) workouts can help us with ghrelin regulation. Focusing on improving diet (and eating enough), choosing the right form of exercise, getting a good night's sleep, and reducing stress can have a profound impact on our weight.

Now about that estrogen dominance...what can we do to find balance? When you consider what we reviewed about endocrine disruptors and all of the xenoestrogens we encounter on a daily basis, I believe we should do what we can to avoid these extra estrogens. If you are like I was prior to doing 16-plus years of research on endocrine disruptors, then you may still be unknowingly consuming or exposing yourself to these xenoestrogens every day. We need to consider the foods we are eating, the personal care and cleaning products we are using, the water we are drinking, what we are storing or cooking our food in, along with reducing stress (which spikes our cortisol, starting the rollercoaster ride). This means we will need to choose foods without all the added hormones and pesticides/fertilizers whenever possible to reduce our body burden of these endocrine disruptors. I know these foods are typically higher in cost, but when you consider both the long-term health benefits and the effect it will have on your hormones and weight...trust me, it's worth it! Next, we are looking into full house water filters that help to remove the unwanted endocrine disruptors...because we don't just drink the water, we shower and bathe ourselves in it, too. However, even if you are unable to install a full house water filter, there are smaller steps and options that you can take to reduce your exposure. I would recommend investigating all of your options to get the cleanest water possible. As far as personal care and cleaning products, it's best to replace all of the toxic-filled products with products that won't harm you or your family. Our family totally pitched (or ditched) all of the products filled with yucky stuff and opted for products we don't have to worry about!!! Other changes we have made is trying to reduce the use of plastic, including where we store our leftovers. Plus, we bake and cook in either glass or stainless steel dishes/pots. Lastly, I want to share an extra step that I am taking...as I was encouraged by my integrative medicine doctor. I am scheduled to discuss the removal of some partial mercury fillings in my mouth in less than two weeks. So, depending on the timing of the release of this book, I may have already had them removed. However, this is just another step in my process to remove all the remaining endocrine disruptors that I am constantly exposed to. Keep in mind that I have been on this journey for many years, and I have gradually made the changes listed above as I learned about the impact they were having on my health. Unfortunately, because these toxins bioaccumulate in our bodies, we also have to take steps to flush them out of our system. However, the most important step we can take is to avoid exposure. This is a vital step if we want to find balance...and find our optimal...and our spunk! We can try to ignore the fact that these xenoestrogens are having an effect on us, but we would only be lying to ourselves and setting ourselves up for future issues/imbalances. The choice is in your hands! YOU have the power to make a difference with your health...what will you choose?

Staying on top of all of our hormones is key. Our body is a system...so if anything is off, it doesn't just affect that hormone or one specific area of the body, it affects the entire body system. Therefore, it's important to figure out the root cause of your symptoms so that you can take action steps. I would highly encourage you to follow the preventative steps whether you are currently experiencing symptoms or not. However, if you are experiencing symptoms, seek out an integrative or functional medicine doctor that can help you find the root cause. For some, it may be a simple solution, but others may need to dig deeper into checking other hormone levels, or additional testing may be required. For instance conditions such as Candida, a virus (e.g., Epstein Barr Virus), or MTHFR gene may cause you to have additional issues that require assistance. Our goal is to find balance, but we also need to find the root cause of our issues. It doesn't do any good to treat a symptom without knowing what is at the root of it all. Are you ready to ditch the imbalances and find balance? Good...me too!

Chapter 8

Ditch the Low Energy

Do you struggle with low energy? Do you wish you could lay down and take an afternoon nap every day? Would you rather skip an evening event so that you can go home and just rest? If you are constantly feeling drained and have no energy, then I would say it's time to do a little investigating to uncover the cause. Is something consistently causing you to lose sleep? Do you have a sluggish thyroid? Unhealthy gut? Overtaxed liver? Adrenal fatigue? Whatever the cause, nobody likes to feel overwhelmed by tiredness all of the time.

Do you feel like you need caffeine to make it through your day? Or, do you feel like not even caffeine seems to give you the energy that you need? If you feel this way, then it's definitely time to find some energy...without caffeine! Have you ever done a cleanse and then noticed you have increased energy? It's no wonder with everything that we have discussed that can bog down our systems that we end up drained for energy. Our liver ends up spending the majority of its time trying to process and detox all of the extra toxins and xenoestrogens that are overloading our system. Plus, food intolerances and too much bad bacteria in our guts cause us to feel tired and sluggish.

We will talk about common ways to naturally increase energy along with suggestions based off of what I have discussed in the preceding chapter. However, I also want to talk about our mitochondria. Have you heard of them? Do you know what they are, what they do, and why they are important? Mitochondria are considered organelles, and they are housed within almost every cell in our body. They serve as the primary source of our energy. It is in our mitochondria where food is converted into adenosine triphosphate (ATP), which provides us with energy. So, in a nutshell, our bodies create the majority of our energy from the foods that we eat (and the air that we breathe). Without this energy our bodies wouldn't function well. So, if our mitochondria get damaged or are not functioning properly, we will have less energy and experience increased fatigue, along with other issues.

What causes our mitochondria to run less efficiently, or how do they become damaged? If you do a quick web search, you will come across a ton of journal articles that talk about mitochondria damage and oxidative stress along with research on the benefits of antioxidants. Oxidative stress causes damage to our cells, and it is a result of repeated bad habits. Factors such as smoking, toxin exposure, sunburns, and poor eating habits can play a role in the damage. It's crazy to think that we are slowly creating damage throughout our bodies with oxidative stress! Learning about mitochondria damage really helped me to understand the need for antioxidants.

Okay...now that we have all the negative junk out of the way, let's move on to the positive! How can we gain more energy? Or, rather, what can we do to boost our energy naturally...without all the extra caffeine or energy drinks? Are you ready for more energy?

• • •

FIND YOUR SPUNK TIP:
Avoid Processed Foods and Sugar

• • •

A couple of years ago, I would have considered someone's lack of energy to be either thyroid or adrenal-related. However, when my thyroid labs (with the full panel) kept coming back within a decent range, I realized that something else was causing my issues...so, I first thought of my adrenal glands. When my cortisol levels came back and no big issues were revealed, I had to keep searching...which is what lead me to learn all about the microbiome and the health of our gut/liver. I'm happy I discovered the answers...and thankful for the return of my energy. So, I want to share what has been a big help in restoring my energy.

If you have never had a full-thyroid panel, I would highly recommend getting some additional lab work done. Like I said in the *Ditch the Imbalance* chapter, if one hormone is off, it can throw the other hormones off. So, this is an easy first step to take to make sure all of your thyroid levels are within the optimal range. With T3 being the active thyroid hormone, this is a key level to keep in the optimal range if you want the most energy. As we discussed, our gut/liver health and stress can have an impact on our thyroid level, so it's also important to focus in on all the areas of ditching the junk (as mentioned throughout this book). Ditching the gunk from our gut/liver will also have a HUGE effect on energy levels. I felt a big difference in just one week from switching up my diet (Anti-Candida and Low FODMAP) and adding in healthy fats (especially coconut oil and MCT oil) and Omega-3 fatty acids (like chia and flaxseed...and salmon). My doctor also suggested taking an Omega-3 supplement, that has been and continues to be part of my daily routine. Also, since our liver is the key to a healthy metabolism, we need to give it a little love! A healthy liver will also help support a healthy balance to our hormones, and increase energy to the body. Our liver is responsible for removing excess toxins and hormones from the bloodstream, so it's an important organ to support for our overall health and wellness.

We talked about the importance of resetting our Circadian rhythm, but we didn't address the importance of a good night's sleep. Did you know that sleep is probably the most important thing you can do for your health? Getting the proper amount of sleep can greatly improve all aspects of our health. Plus, as a Speech-Language Pathologist, I learned that sleep was essential for individuals who encounter difficulties such as traumatic brain injury because it's during sleep when the brain begins the healing process. So, it makes sense that sleep would be an important activity for our general health and wellness. The recommended amount of sleep for an adult is between seven and nine hours a night, but it varies depending on the individual (and the quality of sleep). A good night's sleep can have an impact on many aspects of our health and overall performance, including digestive and immune health, and it even affects our weight. So, we need to make sure we're getting the rest we need both for energy and for our overall health.

How do we improve our mitochondria to increase our energy level? Since our mitochondria is damaged by our negative habits, it seems clear that we need to avoid these habits. In addition, one key step we need to take is to reduce our stress. We cannot always eliminate our stressors, but we can choose activities that will help us to decrease our stress levels...but more on that in the upcoming chapter, *Ditch the Stress*. I don't believe many of us realize the amount of stress we deal with on a daily basis and how it is affecting our energy levels. Next, in looking at the factors that negatively impact our mitochondria, we would be best to avoid smoking, toxin exposure, getting sunburns, and poor eating habits. Even overeating can cause issues, so we should be mindful of both what we are eating and how much. We should be eating a healthy diet, rich in healthy fats (including Omega-3s), protein, and fiber...along with a diet rich in antioxidants and phytonutrients...and ditching sugar and processed foods. My omega supplement also contains Coenzyme Q10 (CoQ10), which plays a role in energy production (and is stored in the mitochondria). Additionally, making sure you are drinking plenty of clean water is important, too. Staying hydrated helps us maintain our energy. Plus, considering what we just discussed about our liver, we should consider detoxing our bodies from the myriad of toxins.

Also, provided you don't have any exercise restrictions, exercise can be another source of energy. Exercise plays a key role in helping to improve our mitochondria. I'm not going to bore you with the science behind it all, but the main point is that adaptations occur during exercise that allow for an increase in size and number of mitochondria, which results in better functioning and an increase in energy. Plus, due to the release of epinephrine and norepinephrine when we exercise, we experience an increase in both circulation and metabolism. So, with the beneficial effects exercise has on our mitochondria along with the release of hormones...and stress reliever for some, it can be a key player when we need to boost our energy levels.

I know this has been a lot of information to digest, but I hope you can see that small changes in our diet and routine can reap BIG results with our health...and energy! It's amazing what a healthy, nutrient-dense diet along with a good night's sleep can do to boost energy levels! A full thyroid lab panel is important, too, and can better help you to see what is going on with thyroid functioning. Plus, by taking care of our mitochondria through diet and exercise (and sleep), we will not only experience a boost in energy, but we may see additional benefits (e.g., improved memory and weight loss). Energy plays a huge role in how optimally our bodies function...including how our bodies process toxins from our environment. Therefore, although the entire book is about finding optimal balance and living abundantly, it's kind of hard to find your spunk if you don't have energy.

Chapter 9

Ditch the Stress

STRESS!!! Do you have any idea the level to which stress impacts our weight?! There are so many factors involved with stress. Plus, stress comes in many different forms...and it's not always what we are feeling as far as emotions. We bring on stress from our packed and rushed schedules and by burning the candle at both ends. When we consistently don't get enough sleep, it stresses our bodies. Another factor is inflammation. For example, chronic inflammation in our bodies caused by food intolerances, a poor diet, or by chronic pain (from injury or even a high-intensity workout) are seen as stressors, and our bodies respond in much the same way as if it was an emotional stressor. Even dehydration, not drinking enough water, is stressful for our bodies.

When we are faced with stress, whether internal or external, our adrenal gland releases the hormone cortisol in response to the stress. Cortisol is often referred to as the "stress hormone." It is not by nature a bad hormone because it's a hormone that protects us when we sense or encounter danger. It provides us with the "fight or flight" response, when epinephrine (adrenaline) is released, increasing our heart rate and blood pressure. So, in times of real danger, the release of cortisol is a good thing. The issue arises when our bodies are in a constant state of stress, and cortisol is frequently spiking. Our bodies are meant to only have short periods or bouts of cortisol being released, not a continuous firing of cortisol. The quick episodes allow our bodies to return to a normal state, but a continuous firing will cause stress on our adrenal glands. This, then, potentially leads to decreased output by the adrenals (and coinciding symptoms).

A chronic-stress state not only affects our adrenal glands, but it can wreak havoc on our thyroid, sex hormones, and our body as a whole. The impact even extends to our gut. Stress has been said to kill the bacteria in our guts. Plus, there is a huge interplay with all of our hormones, so as mentioned previously, when one hormone is out of balance it will affect the others in one form or another. For instance, stress has a negative impact on our weight, and we tend to see weight gain in the abdomen area. Plus, we often see an increase in blood sugar levels, trouble with digestion (shutting down or decreasing functioning to focus on "problem"), and a suppressed immune system.

$$\uparrow Cortisol =$$
$$\uparrow Insulin \downarrow Progesterone \downarrow Thyroid$$

I believe most would agree that stress is not good, and that we need to reduce our levels to help us achieve optimal wellness. However, I want to touch a little bit more on how it causes weight gain. Stress can actually shut down our appetite in the short term because when our body is in the "fight or flight" state then our "rest and digest" part of the parasympathetic nervous system is shut down temporarily. However, the continuous state of stress is another story. Cortisol increases our appetites, which can have a negative impact on our waistlines if our cortisol levels don't return to normal. It may affect what types of foods we choose to eat as well. It also appears that highly processed foods decrease the feedback system from the digestive tract to the brain. We tend to crave sweets when we are stressed due to decreased serotonin levels, and sugary foods provide us with a temporary boost of energy by increasing the serotonin in the brain. This is why many refer to the foods we eat in stressful situations, as "comfort food."

I want to break this down another way...because when I started thinking about our system this way, I finally had an 'aha' moment. Our bodies basically have two states that we can be in..."fight or flight" or "rest and digest." We've been talking a lot about what happens when our body is under a lot of stress, or in the "fight or flight" mode; however, let's look more at the opposite state, "rest and digest." If our digestion slows down or shuts down during stress, I think it is safe to say that we should try to avoid eating during times of stress. This is because our body is not going to properly digest the food we eat. When we are in a parasympathetic state of "rest and digest," adrenaline and cortisol levels drop, and we are more relaxed. Our bodies are then able to focus on proper digestion...and healing. This state is critical for our health because we need to be in this stress-free state in order for our body to heal or repair itself. Stress puts us more at risk for gut issues, including ulcers and infections. So, except for those critical moments when the "fight or flight" state is necessary, we need to strive to be in a more relaxed state to allow our body to do necessary functions to help our bodies digest, detox, and heal.

I hope this gives you a basic picture of what happens when our bodies are under constant stress, without spewing too much technical information. However, there is one more piece of information I want to add for my thyroid peeps before we move on. If you're already dealing with stress or adrenal issues, be

Chapter 10

Ditch the Stinkin' Thinkin'

Just don't do it! Negative thoughts and negative self-talk get us nowhere. Well, they actually might take us backwards because this kind of thinking is detrimental to our health. In one of my yoga trainings, they took us through an exercise where we were changing our posture...and then we were told to repeat the same open and closed positions, but with a smile. Would you believe the act of smiling can change how we feel? Go ahead and try it for yourself.

Have you ever felt like conquering the world (or even a small project) when you're feeling like Eeyore? If you're like most, you probably felt like being alone and just doing something to numb the mind and pass the time away. On the other hand, let us pretend you received the best news and you're on cloud nine...are you ready to tackle the world now? My guess is that your view of life, and your ambition to get things done are drastically different in those two situations. So, I ask you, what does it profit you to have stinkin' thinkin'?

Dr. Caroline Leaf, cognitive neuroscientist and author of many books, including *Who Switched Off My Brain?: Controlling Toxic Thoughts and Emotions* and *Switch On Your Brain Workbook: The Key to Peak Happiness, Thinking, and Health,* does an excellent job of explaining the process of what happens inside of our brains when we think positive versus negative thoughts. Positive thoughts help build or regrow the "branches" in our brain, whereas negative thoughts do the opposite. If you've never listened to Dr. Caroline Leaf speak, I highly encourage you to look up her videos on YouTube. She confirms that negative thoughts are toxic and can make us sick. If we want optimal health, then we need to focus our thoughts on what is lovely and pure (positive).

• • •

FIND YOUR SPUNK TIP:
Make a List of All Your Blessings...
Start a Gratitude Journal

• • •

What causes us to have stinkin' thinkin'? What can we do to avoid it, even when life's circumstances seem to be going against us? Years ago, I read the book *Happiness is a Choice* by Frank Minirth, MD and Paul Meier, MD when I was going through a hard time. That book helped me to realize that my situation didn't dictate my feelings; I could choose to be happy regardless of my circumstances. It was probably around that time that I also discovered the Attitude quote by Charles Swindoll that I printed out and taped to my mirror to read every day. The quote is as follows:

"The longer I live, the more I realize the impact of attitude on life.

Attitude, to me, is more important than facts. It is more important than the past, than education, than money, than circumstances, than failures, than successes, than what other people think or say or do. It is more important than appearance, giftedness or skill. It will make or break a company... a church... a home.

The remarkable thing is we have a choice every day regarding the attitude we will embrace for that day. We cannot change our past... we cannot change the fact that people will act in a certain way. We cannot change the inevitable. The only thing we can do is play on the one string we have, and that is our attitude... I am convinced that life is 10% what happens to me and 90% how I react to it.

And so it is with you... we are in charge of our attitudes."

It's empowering to know that we have the power within us to change our attitudes and even our emotional state. In thinking about this concept, it made me think back to one of my college classes on sports psychology. We learned how elite athletes visualize themselves successfully performing at their particular sport to help them increase their chances of winning. So, knowing we are in charge of our attitudes, let's consider some activities we can initiate to begin creating positive habits to keep us from falling into stinkin' thinkin'!

First, I believe we have to daily renew our minds. We have to take action steps every single day to help us stay positive. I find it helpful to place reminders in places that we are likely to look each day (like on the bathroom mirror) to help prompt us to keep our attitudes in check. Another positive action we can put into place is to start each day with an "attitude of gratitude." This is a great way to kick off our day in a positive way. It's hard to be negative when you consider all of the blessings in your life. Next, journaling is a powerful tool to help us express our thoughts and feelings, along with recording daily habits to help us make positive changes. More specifically, for the purpose of changing our way of thinking, a gratitude list or journal is a great way to help us focus on the positive aspects of our lives. So whether you record a list each day of what you're thankful for or you create a gratitude journal, you're making positive steps to change your thinking.

Personally, I find that listening to uplifting music and spending time in prayer help me to let go of the negative and focus on the positive. Plus, I've learned that pure essential oils can have a positive effect on our emotions. Our sense of smell is directly linked to our limbic system, so scents can have a huge impact on our feelings. Have you ever smelled a certain aroma that reminds you of something from your past (positive or negative)? Aromatherapy can have a wonderful effect on our moods. Lastly, spending quality time with family and friends...playing and laughing together is also a favorite activity of mine. Although, I should add an interesting observation about myself before we move on. I have often had people comment about my smile, but I went through a period where I kind of felt my "sparkle" fade. I just lacked the energy to spend time with others...and I noticed a true difference in the way that I felt. Would you believe this was during a time that my thyroid levels were less than optimal? I'm sure gut issues were in play too. Honestly, when your levels (and body system, in general) are out-of-balance, it's hard to pull yourself out of a funk. So, if you are feeling that way, it's time to get to the root cause of your issues...and know that there is hope! So, whether you adopt the ideas that I've listed or have other ways that have proven to help you keep a positive attitude, put these into practice daily. I believe our way of thinking will either hinder or heal us. Imagine yourself having optimal wellness.

Chapter 11

My Biggest Game Changers

Can you believe we are almost done?! I have enjoyed sharing my journey and the things that I have learned with you, but now I want to take time to break it all down, so that I can list out the key steps that I took to find my optimal...my spunk. I would encourage you to read over everything again to fully digest it all; however, this chapter will be an easy reference guide to help you put it all together. Are you ready to break it all down and weed through all the extra details? These were my biggest game changers...and my suggestions for you. I am not a physician...and although I have learned a lot as a certified health coach and personal trainer (and even some as a Speech-Language Pathologist), these tips are based off of my personal experience of living almost seventeen years without a thyroid. I offer these suggestions as a gift, in hopes that you will not have to endure the trials that I have had to experience these past several years. Many times I have wished that I would have learned all of this information years ago...but I cannot change the past, I can only move forward. So, I offer you these valuable tools that I have learned. May they prove to be a blessing in your life...and if so, don't forget to pass the blessing on to someone else.

My biggest game changer tips:

Be your own advocate! Remember that you know your body better than anyone. Doctors can treat symptoms, but at what cost? Make sure you find the root cause of your issues. If you focus on treating symptoms and never discover the true cause, then you are just setting yourself up for a continuous cycle of treating symptoms.

Request a full thyroid panel and corresponding labs. It's helpful to get a complete picture of what is going on with your thyroid levels, along with lab tests that often go hand-in-hand with thyroid disease. A good thyroid panel will include the following: TSH, Free T4, Free T3, Reverse T3, and antibody labs. Typical corresponding labs include: B12, Iron panel, and Vitamin D. Also, make sure you have a practitioner who is willing to help you find your optimal level...which may include looking at other factors beyond increasing thyroid medicine (and choose natural thyroid solutions whenever possible).

DITCH the endocrine disruptors!!! If you want to find balance with your thyroid and ALL of your hormones, it's vital that you do whatever you can to avoid these disruptors. Prevention is always the best route. Choose foods, water, and products that don't contain all of the endocrine disruptors. Read labels...know what you are using! Do a little research of your own and learn about the ingredients in the products that you have been using. Consume and use foods/products without all the yuck, as much as possible!

Test for food intolerances. Do testing or an elimination diet to determine any food intolerances...and then remove them from your diet. Also, remember that there is a reason for the food intolerances, and you will also need to figure out the root cause. For me, it was Candida (and coinciding SIBO) which created a leaky gut...leading to histamine intolerance with these food intolerances. I started with an Anti-Candida diet using mainly foods on a Low FODMAP diet. Removing these foods is extremely important for the healing process! If you don't remove them it's like adding insult to injury.

The key foods that I removed were:

- Peanuts
- Oats
- Corn
- Gluten
- Dairy
- Soy
- Eggs
- Sugar

Other foods to be mindful of are antinutrients, which can be found in beans, seeds, raw cruciferous veggies, etc. Try soaking beans and seeds, cooking cruciferous veggies, and fermenting foods to reduce the effects. Additionally, be mindful of processed foods, caffeine, coffee, and alcohol consumption. It might be hard, but you can do it!

Use a food journal. If you choose to do an elimination diet, make sure to use a food journal. This will allow you to keep track of what you are eating along with symptoms you may experience...keeping in mind that food intolerance symptoms can occur up to 72 hours later. So, make sure you keep track of the day and time that you ate a particular food...and only add one food back in at a time. It is also helpful to make a note of your general feelings when eating certain foods. Of course, food journaling can also help you stay on track and keep track of key nutrients, like protein, fats, and carbs. I also find it helpful to track my water intake as well.

Find a diet that works for you! After you have removed any food intolerances and any antinutrients that seem to cause issues, choose a plan that works best for you. I would, however, recommend avoiding artificial and processed foods, along with sugar...or anything that turns to sugar!!! Plus, I believe that healthy fats should be an essential part of our diets because they are vital for optimal brain and body functioning. Oh, and don't forget your veggies!!! As I mentioned earlier in the book, I tend to follow more of a Paleoish, healthy Keto-cycling type diet with some intermittent fasting. I have definitely increased my healthy fats and veggies, especially sulfur-rich veggies. I use MCT oil in my morning shakes and use a variety of healthy oils (e.g., coconut, olive, MCT, avocado, and macadamia) on my veggies every single day. I have honestly never tested for ketones because I'm not a strict diet follower...just try to eat healthy. If your liver and thyroid are functioning optimally then your body should be fairly metabolically flexible. So, you need to figure out what is right for YOU!

Eat Pre- and Probiotic Rich Foods! Hippocrates, the father of western medicine, nailed it on the head when he said, "All disease begins in the gut." The health of our guts is one of the keys to abundant living!!! Our gut health can affect more than just our physical health. It has the potential to affect our brain health, emotions, and mental state as well. We need to do everything we can to build a strong and healthy microbiome. Our gut flora is like our inner garden...and you know what happens to a garden that is not well-cared for - it is overtaken by weeds! So, feeding our gut phytonutrient-rich foods along with foods that feed the good bacteria is essential for a healthy gut. Chapter six had a lot of information that I'm not going to repeat, but just make sure you go back and read all of the suggestions for helping to restore a healthy gut and liver.

Find balance. Balance is an important part of learning to thrive. We need balance in our daily schedule and habits (especially eating and sleeping) as well as for our hormones. Start with the easy tasks you can implement on your own, and everything might start to balance on their own. However, it is important to figure out what is at the root of the imbalance...don't just take a pill to "treat" a symptom expecting that it is going to solve the problem. I've learned that we can be too quick with upping our thyroid medication, too, if our Free T3 levels come back less than optimal. First, figure out what is causing the low T3. For instance, is it your diet (e.g., Keto) or is there a gut/liver issue? Amazingly, a lot of our issues can be resolved by simple tweaks in our lifestyle and diet. I have personally adjusted my sleeping and eating habits to be more in line with the suggested pattern to help reset my Circadian Rhythm. The cool part of it all is that I no longer need an alarm clock to wake up...which means my body wakes up when it's ready! Balance equals peace of mind...and body.

Find your energy! Key areas to look at are thyroid levels, adrenal health, liver health, and mitochondria. Again, make sure to do a full thyroid panel and check adrenal functioning, if necessary. Plus, follow all the tips for finding balance, too...especially getting plenty of sleep. Following a diet to improve both my gut and liver health was key to finding my spunk. The biggest game changers for me were removing the food intolerances and sugar (and of course, no processed foods), being careful not to overeat, eating when not stressed (taking deep breaths...and praying before my meal), eating and drinking foods/drinks that were rich in phytonutrients (and antioxidants)...and clean, filtered water, and adding in plenty of healthy oils (especially coconut and MCT), fermented veggies, probiotic water, prebiotics (including resistant starches), Omega-3s (flaxseeds, chia seeds, hemp seed, and salmon), and probiotics. Lastly, I continue to maintain an exercise routine. Finding the right balance of healthy, nutrient-dense foods (with some additional supplements) along with exercise and a good night's sleep can revive your energy levels and put a little pep in your step!

Reduce stress...create oxytocin!!! Take a deep breath...relax...hug someone. No really...it's truly that simple! Find what you enjoy most and do it. When we find our "happy place" we allow our parasympathetic nervous system to properly rest and digest. Try to incorporate activities such as yoga, prayer and/or meditation, spending time with friends, deep breathing, listening to music, being grateful, smiling, laughing, playing, or hugging a friend/family member. I like to do many of these activities and I've been intentional about making sure to get at least eight hugs a day. So, figure out activities that are calming for you...and make a point to find joy in every day. Find someone to hug! Yes, go do it!!!

Adopt a positive mindset. Start your day with listing three to five things for which you are grateful. It's amazing what a difference it can make in your day when you start it with thinking about your blessings. Post reminders around your house, like on your bathroom mirror, if needed. Remember that happiness is a choice, and you have the power to set your mood for the day. Consider buying a journal to use as a gratitude journal and add your grateful list along with any other blessings in your life. Personally, I am thankful for each day that God allows me to wake up for another day. I also try to find the hidden blessing in the hard moments, too. Lastly, your brain believes what you tell it, so make sure you speak life to yourself. Choose positive talk and eliminate all of the negative self-talk from your vocabulary. Believe in yourself and claim the positive words you speak over your life. A positive mindset is the icing on the cake.

I hope that you are able to take all of my biggest game changers and apply them to your life and circumstances. We all have different genetics; however, I believe most of the tips that I have shared can benefit everyone...they are not exclusive to me! These are strategies that can make a big impact if you choose to implement them. It is my hope and prayer that my experiences (especially the difficult ones I have endured) will make a positive difference in your life...or for someone you love. I hope that you have learned something new and that it ends up being a blessing in your life. My true desire for you is that you are able to 'find your spunk'!

Appendix A

Additional Information on Endocrine Disruptors

Introduction to Endocrine Disrupting Chemicals (EDCs): A Guide for Public Interest Organizations and Policy-Makers.
www.endocrine.org/-/media/endosociety/files/advocacy-and-outreach/important-documents/introduction-to-endocrine-disrupting-chemicals.pdf?la=en

Endocrine Disruptors.
Information from the National Institute of Environmental Health Sciences on Endocrine Disruptors.
https://www.niehs.nih.gov/health/materials/endocrine_disruptors_508.pdf

Fluoride and Your Thyroid
https://stopthethyroidmadness.com/fluoride-and-your-thyroid/

Neurobehavioural Effects of Developmental Toxicity.
https://www.thelancet.com/journals/laneur/article/PIIS1474-4422%2813%2970278-3/fulltext#article_upsell

Dirty Dozen Endocrine Disruptors
Environmental Working Group's Dirty Dozen list and explanation of the top endocrine disruptors to avoid: https://www.ewg.org/research/dirty-dozen-list-endocrine-disruptors.

3 Lesser Known Sources of Fluoride Harming Your Thyroid
Dr. Alan Christianson: https://youtu.be/rFVTUNZN7Pk

Appendix B

Recommended Labs & Optimal Lab Values

A full thyroid panel typically includes the following labs:
- TSH (yes, we still look at this value)
- Free T4
- Free T3
- Reverse T3

If Hashimoto's is suspected:
- Thyroid Peroxidase Antibodies (TPOAb)
- Thyroglobulin Antibodies (TgAb)

If Grave's Disease is suspected:
- Thyroid Receptor Antibodies (TRAb)
- Thyroid Stimulating Immunoglobulins (TSI)

If Thyroid Cancer is suspected:
- Thyroglobulin (Tg)

Key Corresponding Labs:

- Iron Panel (Ferritin, Iron Saturation, TIBC [Total Iron Binding Capacity], Total Serum)
- Vitamin B12
- Vitamin D
- Comprehensive Metabolic Panel (Magnesium, Sodium, Potassium)

For more information, including additional labs that are beneficial, check out the following links:

- http://www.thyroidchange.org/testing.html
- https://stopthethyroidmadness.com/recommended-labwork/

ORDER YOUR OWN LABS!!!

YourLabWork Link: https://yourlabwork.com/?ref=677

Can't find a doctor who will order a full-thyroid panel...or you just want to order your own labs. Use my affiliate link to receive discounted labs (at 50-80% less than you would pay elsewhere) in a safe, confidential and convenient way.

Note: I am not a medical doctor and I cannot receive lab results from the lab, read or interpret labs, or diagnose or treat any medical conditions. However, what I can do is share with you Dr. Alan Hopkins' optimal functional ranges for labs, guide you to resources to help you understand your labs; share with you food, lifestyle, and supplements you may want to consider based on your lab results and share anything I see that raises potential concerns or red flags that you may want to investigate further or discuss with your doctor.

Optimal Lab Values:

Due to the slight variance in the suggested optimal lab values, I have provided a couple of links for your review. The key is to look at the optimal levels...NOT "normal!"

Dr. Alan Christianson:
- drchristianson.com/how-to-test-your-thyroid-the-definitive-guide
- Thyroid Lab Analyzer: thyroidlabanalyzer.com

Thyroid Nation:
- https://thyroidnation.com/thyroid-lab-tests-telling-truth/

Stop The Thyroid Madness (STTM):
- stopthethyroidmadness.com/lab-values

Appendix C

Additional Resources

RESOURCES MENTIONED IN BOOK:

30 Amazing Resistant Starch Foods for Better Digestion
Dr. Alan Christianson (2018)
https://drchristianson.com/30-amazing-resistant-starch-foods-for-better-digestion/

Identification of the 100 Richest Dietary Sources of Polyphenols: An Application of the Phenol-Explorer Database.
Pérez-Jiménez, J., Neveu, V., Vos, F., & Scalbert, A. (Published: 2010, November 3).
European Journal of Clinical Nutrition volume 64, pages S112–S120 (2010). https://www.nature.com/articles/ejcn2010221

Common Symptoms of Thyroid Disease:

- **Hypothyroidism symptoms:**
  https://www.endocrineweb.com/conditions/hypothyroidism/symptoms-hypothyroidism

- **Hyperthyroidism symptoms:**
  https://www.endocrineweb.com/conditions/hyperthyroidism/hyperthyroidism-symptoms

- **Thyroid Disease Symptoms Checklist:**
  https://www.holtorfmed.com/wp-content/uploads/2017/12/ ThyroidChecklist.pdf

Elimination Diet Protocol Options

The premise behind an elimination diet is the same, but there are variations as far as which foods to eat or remove. Here are a couple elimination diet protocols that focus on removing foods that cause inflammation:

- The Autoimmune Protocol (AIP)
- Low-FODMAP

MORE HELPFUL RESOURCES:

Best Salt Options:
- Celtic Sea Salt (Selina Naturally)
- Himalayan Salt
- Real Salt (Sea Salt by Redmond)

For additional resources, including an example of my daily food/supplement routine, my favorite household and personal products, my recommendations for best deals on organic products and clean, grass-fed meats, and a link to my *Ditch the Junk, Find Your Spunk: Food & Gratitude Journal* go to: **www.swfitnut.com/findyourspunk**.

Also, to make it easier for you, I have included all of the previous resource links at **www.swfitnut.com/findyourspunk**.

Appendix D

My Favorite People/Pages to Follow

Dr. Alan Christianson, NMD
drchristianson.com
Social links:
Facebook: www.facebook.com/DrAlanChristianson
Instagram: @dralanchristianson
Books: *The Metabolism Reset Diet; The Adrenal Reset Diet; The Complete Idiot's Guide to Thyroid Health*

Dr. Amy Myers, MD
www.amymyersmd.com
Social links:
Facebook: www.facebook.com/AmyMyersMD
Instagram: @amymyersmd
Books: *The Autoimmune Solution; The Autoimmune Solution Cookbook; The Thyroid Connection*

Dr. Mark Hyman, MD

drhyman.com
Social links:
Facebook: m.facebook.com/drmarkhyman
Instagram/Twitter: @drmarkhyman
Books: *Food: What the Heck Should I Eat?; Eat Fat, Get Thin; The Blood Sugar Solution; 10-Day Detox Diet*

Dr. Sara Gottfried, MD

Website: www.saragottfriedmd.com
Social links:
Facebook: www.facebook.com/DrGottfried
Instagram: @saragottfriedmd
Books: *The Hormone Cure; The Hormone Reset Diet, Brain Body Diet; Younger*

Dr. Joseph Mercola, DO

Website: mercola.com
Social links:
Facebook: www.facebook.com/doctor.health &
www.facebook.com/ Doctor.Salud
Instagram: @drmercola
Books: *KetoFast; Fat for Fuel; Superfuel, Effortless Healing; Take Control of your Health; Sweet Deception; The No-Grain Diet* (and many more….)

Donna Gates, M.Ed, ABAAHP

www.bodyecology.com
Social links:
Facebook: m.facebook.com/BodyEcology
Instagram: @donnamgates & @bodyecologyofficial
Books: *The Body Ecology Diet; Body Ecology Living Cookbook; The Body Ecology Guide to Growing Younger; The Baby Boomer Diet*

JJ Virgin, CNS, CHFS
Website: jjvirgin.com
Social links:
Facebook: m.facebook.com/JJVirginOfficial
Instagram: @jj.virgin
Books: *The Virgin Diet; JJ Virgin's Sugar Impact Diet; The Virgin Diet Cookbook; JJ Virgin's Sugar Impact Diet Cookbook; Warrior Mom* (and many more)

Dr. Josh Axe, DC, DNM, CNS
Website: DrAxe.com
Social links:
Facebook: www.facebook.com/DrJoshAxe
Instagram: @drjoshaxe
Books: *Keto Diet; Eat Dirt; Essential Oils; The Gut Repair Cookbook; The Real Food Diet Cookbook*

Dr. David Jockers, DNM, DC, MS
Website: drjockers.com
Social links:
Facebook: www.facebook.com/DrDavidJockers
Instagram: @drjockers
Books: *SuperCharge Your Brain; SuperCharged Healthy Recipe Book*

Dr. Anna Cabeca, DO, OBGYN, FACOG
Website: drannacabeca.com
Social links:
Facebook: www.facebook.com/Drannac
Instagram: @drannacabeca
Book: *The Hormone Fix*

Chris Kresser, M.S., L.Ac
Website: chriskresser.com
Social links:
Facebook: www.facebook.com/chriskresserlac
Instagram: @chriskresser
Books: *Unconventional Medicine; The Paleo Cure; Your Personal Paleo Code*

Dr. Ben Lynch, ND
Website: drbenlynch.com
Social links:
Facebook: m.facebook.com/drbenjaminlynch
Instagram: @drbenlynch
Book: *Dirty Genes*

Dr. Izabella Wentz, PharmD.
thyroidpharmacist.com
Social links:
Facebook: www.facebook.com/ThyroidLifestyle
Instagram: @izabellawentzpharmd
Books: *Hashimoto's Protocol; Hashimoto's The Root Cause*

Dr. David Perlmutter, MD
Website: drperlmutter.com
Social links:
Facebook: m.facebook.com/DavidPerlmutterMd
Instagram: @davidperlmutter
Books: *Grain Brain; The Grain Brain Whole Life Plan; Brain Maker; Power Up Your Brain; Effortless Healing: Raise a Smarter Child by Kindergarten*

Dr. Eric Berg, DC
Website: drberg.com
Social links:
Facebook: www.facebook.com/drericberg
Instagram: @drericberg
Books: *The New Body Type Guide; The 7 Principles of Fat Burning*

Thomas DeLauer
Website: thomasdelauer.com
Social links:
Facebook: m.facebook.com/thomas.delauer
Instagram: @thomasdelauer
Books: *The Superfood Detox Code; Top 10 Intermittent Fasting Hacks*

Dave Asprey
Website: www.bulletproof.com
Social links:
Facebook: www.facebook.com/bulletproofexecutive & www.facebook.com/ Bulletproof
Instagram: @dave.asprey & @bulletproof
Books: *Super Human; Game Changers; Head Strong; The Bulletproof Diet; Bulletproof: The Cookbook; Upgraded Chef*

Dr. Caroline Leaf, PhD, BSc
Website: drleaf.com
Social links:
Facebook: m.facebook.com/drleaf
Instagram: @drcarolineleaf
Books: *Think, Learn, Succeed; Switch On Your Brain Every Day; Switch On Your Brain; The Perfect You; Think & Eat Yourself Smart; Who Switched Off Your Brain; The Gift in You*

THYROID WEBSITE/PAGES

Thyroid Sexy (Gena Lee Nolin)
Facebook: www.facebook.com/thyroidsexy
Instagram: @thyroid_sexy
Book: *Beautiful Inside & Out*

Mary Shomon's Thyroid Support
Website: www.verywellhealth.com/thyroid-4014636 &
www.mary-shomon.com
Facebook: www.facebook.com/thyroidsupport
Books: *The Menopause Thyroid Solution; The Thyroid Hormone Breakthrough; Living Well with Hypothyroidism; Living Well with Grave's Disease and Hyperthyroidism; Thyroid Guide to Hair Loss; Living Well with Autoimmune Disease; Living Well with Chronic Fatigue Syndrome and Fibromyalgia*

Stop The Thyroid Madness (STTM) (Janie Bowthorpe)
Website: stopthethyroidmadness.com
Facebook: www.facebook.com/StoptheThyroidMadness

ThyroidChange
Website: thyroidchange.org
Facebook: www.facebook.com/ThyroidChange
Instagram: @thyroidchange

Thyroid Nation
Website: www.thyroidnation.com
Facebook: www.facebook.com/thyroidnation1
Instagram: @thyroidnation

References

Bowthorpe, J. (2006, August 21). *Fluoride and your Thyroid—a dangerous connection.* Retrieved from https://stopthethyroidmadness.com/fluoride-and-your-thyroid/

Bulletproof (2015, September 21). *Dr. Sara Gottfried - Your Estrogen Cure: Estrobolome & Rock Star Ratios - 2014 Bulletproof Conference.* Retrieved from https://youtu.be/38Ueovkogq0

Cabeca, A. (2019). *A Ketogenic Diet Optimized for Thyroid Health.* Retrieved from https://drannacabeca.com/blogs/keto-alkaline-diet/a-ketogenic-diet-optimized-for-thyroid-health

Cabeca, A. (n.d.). *Put More Oxytocin into Your Life for a Healthier You.* Retrieved from https://drannacabeca.com/blogs/hormone-imbalance/put-more-oxytocin-into-your-life-for-a-healthier-you

Christianson, A. (2014, November 25 Published). *Curing Cortisol with Carbs – Dr. Alan Christianson*. Retrieved from https://www.saragottfriedmd.com/curing-cortisol-with-carbs-dr-alan-christianson/

Christianson, A. (2019). *The Metabolism Reset Diet*. New York: Harmony Books.

Costantini, L., Molinari, R., Farinon, B., Merendino, N. (2017). *Impact of Omega-3 Fatty Acids on the Gut Microbiota*. International Journal of Molecular Science, 18(12) 2645. doi: 10.3390/ijms18122645 Retrieved from: https://www.ncbi.nlm.nih.gov/pmc/articles/PMC5751248/

Gates, D. (2011). *The Body Ecology Diet: Recovering Your Health and Rebuilding Your Immunity*. Carlsbad, CA: Hay House, Inc.

Gates, D. (2014, Mar 7). *Understanding Gut Health: The Root of All Wellness In the Kitchen w/ JJ Virgin-Donna-Body Ecology*. Retrieved from https://youtu.be/S6Pdsryqb8o

Gore, A.C., Crews, D., Doan, L.L., La Merrill, M. and Zota, A. (2014, December). *Introduction to Endocrine Disrupting Chemicals (EDCs): A Guide for Public Interest Organizations and Policy-Makers*. Retrieved from https://www.endocrine.org/-/media/endosociety/files/advocacy-and-outreach/important-documents/introduction-to-endocrine-disrupting-chemicals.pdf?la=en

References

Higgins, J. A. (2015, January 1). *Critical Review Food Science Nutrition* Retrieved from https://www.ncbi.nlm.nih.gov/pmc/articles/PMC4220782/

Kshirsagar, S. (2018, January 9). *Yoga, Aryuveda & Lifestyle Medicine: The Amazing Healing Power of Daily Habits.* Downloaded from YogaUOnline.com.

Myers, A. (2018, April 3). *3 Important Reasons to Give Up Gluten if You Have an Autoimmune Disease.* Retrieved from https://www.amymyersmd.com/2018/04/3-reasons-give-up-gluten-autoimmune-disease/

Myers, A. (2019). *9 Causes of Estrogen Dominance and What to Do About It.* Retrieved from https://www.amymyersmd.com/2019/03/9-causes-estrogen-dominance/

Michaels, J. (2009). *Master Your Metabolism: The 3 DIET Secrets to Naturally Balancing Your Hormones for a Hot and Healthy Body.* New York, NY: Crown Publishers.

Minirith, F.B. and Meier, P.D. (1978). *Happiness is a Choice: A Manual on the Symptoms, Causes, and Cures of Depression.* Grand Rapids, MI: Baker Books.

Pérez-Jiménez, J., Neveu, V., Vos, F., & Scalbert, A. (Published: 2010, November 3).*Identification of the 100 richest dietary sources of polyphenols: an application of the Phenol-Explorer database*. European Journal of Clinical Nutrition volume 64, pages S112–S120 (2010). Retrieved from: https://www.nature.com/ articles/ejcn2010221

Ratini, M. (2017, November 23). *Can Coffee Help Your Liver?* Retrieved from https://www.webmd.com/hepatitis/coffee-help-liver#2

Shamblin, G. (1997). *The Weigh Down Diet*. New York, NY: Doubleday.

Shomon, M. (2009). *The Thyroid Menopause Solution: Overcome Menopause by Solving Your Hidden Thyroid Problems*. New York, NY: HarperCollins Publishers.

Society for Endocrinology (2019, November 19). *Is the Gut or Brain More Important in Regulating Appetite and Metabolism?*. NeuroscienceNews. Retrieved November 19, 2019 from http://neurosciencenews.com/gut-brain-appetite-10218/

Virgin, J. (2012). *The Virgin Diet: Drop 7 Foods, Lose 7 Pounds, Just 7 Days*. New York, NY: HarperCollins Publishers.

Virgin, J. (2014). *JJ Virgin's Sugar Impact Diet: Drop 7 Hidden Sugars, Lose Up to 10 Pounds in Just 2 Weeks*. New York, NY: Hachette Book Group, Inc.

About the Author

Shellby Winget, SLP, CHC, CPT is a thyroid cancer survivor who has overcome many challenges over the past several years. Her personal experiences led her to search for answers that set her on a more natural, holistic path. She is a thyroid advocate and has a passion for helping others thrive in all areas of their lives (physical, mental, and spiritual). Shellby is on a mission to teach others about the importance of removing toxic chemicals from their homes and personal care products, along with teaching the value of pure essential oils. Plus, she never tires of learning more about nutrition and hormone health. Shellby is the founder of *FIT with Shellby* and offers limited online health coaching services.

Shellby chose to "retire" as a Speech-Language Pathologist and dive into the world of health and fitness. She is currently an online health coach and personal trainer. She holds a M.A. in Communication Sciences (Speech-Language Pathology) from the University of Cincinnati and a B.S. in Psychology and Physical Education from Anderson University. She holds the following certifications from the American Council on Exercise: Health Coach, Personal Trainer, and Group Fitness Instructor. Additionally, Shellby has taken several live YogaFit trainings to gain knowledge on restorative exercises, including *Anatomy & Alignment*, *YogaBack*, *YogaFit Props*, and *Restoring Balance: Training the PNS (Parasympathetic Nervous System)*.

On a personal note, Shellby is a wife and mother. She loves spending time with her family and going on fun adventures. Shellby is constantly sharing her knowledge with friends and family and hopes to instill the value of healthy eating and toxic-free living with her boys.

For more information, please visit Shellby at www.swfitnut.com.

Find me on social media:

facebook/com/coachshellby
instagram.com/coachshellby
twitter.com/coachshellby
linkedin.com/in/shellby-winget